T0362209

Applied Translational Research in Foot and Ankle Surgery

Editor

DONALD D. ANDERSON

FOOT AND ANKLE CLINICS

www.foot.theclinics.com

Consulting Editor
CESAR DE CESAR NETTO

March 2023 • Volume 28 • Number 1

ELSEVIER

1600 John F. Kennedy Boulevard • Suite 1800 • Philadelphia, Pennsylvania, 19103-2899

http://www.theclinics.com

FOOT AND ANKLE CLINICS Volume 28, Number 1
March 2023 ISSN 1083-7515, ISBN-978-0-323-93851-8

Editor: Megan Ashdown
Developmental Editor: Arlene B. Campos

Foot and Ankle Clinics (ISSN 1083-7515) is published quarterly by Elsevier, Inc., 360 Park Avenue South, New York, NY 10010-1710. Months of issue are March, June, September, and December. Periodicals postage paid at New York, NY, and additional mailing offices. Subscription price per year is $362.00 (US individuals), $635.00 (US institutions), $100.00 (US students), $389.00 (Canadian individuals), $762.00 (Canadian institutions), $100.00 (Canadian students), $504.00 (international individuals), $762.00 (international institutions), and $215.00 (international students). To receive student/resident rate, orders must be accompanied by name of affiliated institution, date of term, and the *signature* of program/residency coordinator on institution letterhead. Orders will be billed at individual rate until proof of status is received. Foreign air speed delivery is included in all *Clinics* subscription prices. All prices are subject to change without notice. **POSTMASTER:** Send address changes to *Foot and Ankle Clinics*, Elsevier Health Sciences Division, Subscription Customer Service, 3251 Riverport Lane, Maryland Heights, MO 63043. **Customer Service: 1-800-654-2452 (US and Canada). From outside of the United States and Canada, call 314-447-8871. Fax: 314-447-8029. E-mail: JournalsCustomerService-usa@ elsevier.com (for print support); JournalsOnlineSupport-usa@elsevier.com (for online support).**

Reprints. For copies of 100 or more, of articles in this publication, please contact the Commercial Reprints Department, Elsevier Inc., 360 Park Avenue South, New York, NY 10010-1710. Tel.: 212-633-3874; Fax: 212-633-3820; E-mail: reprints@elsevier.com.

Contributors

CONSULTING EDITOR

CE3AR DE CE3AR NETTO, MD, PhD
Assistant Professor, Director of the Orthopedic Functional Imaging Research Laboratory (OFIRL), Department of Orthopedics and Rehabilitation, University of Iowa, Iowa City, Iowa, USA

EDITOR

DONALD D. ANDERSON, PhD
Professor and Vice Chair of Research, Department of Orthopedics and Rehabilitation, Richard and Jan Johnston Chair in Orthopedic Biomechanics, Professor, Departments of Biomedical Engineering and Industrial and Systems Engineering, The University of Iowa, Iowa City, Iowa, USA

AUTHORS

DONALD D. ANDERSON, PhD
Professor and Vice Chair of Research, Department of Orthopedics and Rehabilitation, Richard and Jan Johnston Chair in Orthopedic Biomechanics, Professor, Departments of Biomedical Engineering and Industrial and Systems Engineering, The University of Iowa, Iowa City, Iowa, USA

CHLOE BARATTA, BS
J. Crayton Pruitt Family Department of Biomedical Engineering, University of Florida, Gainesville, Florida, USA

PAULA R. BECKENKAMP, PhD, BPthy (Hons)
Senior Lecturer, Sydney School of Health Sciences, Faculty of Medicine and Health, The University of Sydney, Camperdown, Sydney, Australia

ADAM D. BITTERMAN, DO
Chairman, Donald and Barbara Zucker School of Medicine at Hofstra/Northwell, Hempstead, New York, USA; Department of Orthopaedic Surgery, Northwell Health—Huntington Hospital, Huntington, New York, USA

CLAIRE BROCKETT, PhD
Professor, Department of Mechanical Engineering, INSIGNEO Institute for in silico Medicine, University of Sheffield, United Kingdom

BRIAN L. DAVIS, PhD
Center for Human Machine Systems, Cleveland State University, Cleveland, Ohio, USA

CLAIRE E. HILLER, PhD, MAppSc, BAppSc
Associate Professor,. Sydney School of Health Sciences, Faculty of Medicine and Health, The University of Sydney, Camperdown, Sydney, Australia

KAREN M. KRUGER, PhD
Motion Analysis Center, Shriners Children's Chicago, Chicago, Illinois, USA; Orthopedic and Rehabilitation Engineering Center, Marquette University and Medical College of Wisconsin, Milwaukee, Wisconsin, USA

JOSEPH J. KRZAK, PT, PhD
Motion Analysis Center, Shriners Children's Chicago, Chicago, Illinois, USA; Physical Therapy Program, Midwestern University, College of Health Sciences, Downers Grove, Illinois, USA

MATTHIEU LALEVÉE, MD, MSc
CETAPS EA3832, Research Center for Sports and Athletic Activities Transformations, University of Rouen Normandy, Mont-Saint-Aignan, France; Department of Orthopedic Surgery, Rouen University Hospital, Rouen, France

LEONARD DANIEL LATT, MD, PhD
Department of Orthopaedic Surgery, University of Arizona, Tucson, Arizona, USA

WILLIAM R. LEDOUX, PhD
Center for Limb Loss and MoBility (CLiMB), VA Puget Sound Health Care System; Departments of Mechanical Engineering and Orthopaedics & Sports Medicine, University of Washington, Seattle, Washington, USA

AMY L. LENZ, PhD
Department of Orthopaedics, University of Utah, Salt Lake City, Utah, USA

RICH J. LISONBEE, MS
Department of Orthopaedics, University of Utah, Salt Lake City, Utah, USA

HAMED MALAKOUTIKHAH, PhD
Department of Aerospace and Mechanical Engineering, University of Arizona, Tucson, Arizona, USA

JESSI K. MARTIN, BS
Center for Human Machine Systems, Cleveland State University, Cleveland, Ohio, USA

JENNIFER A. NICHOLS, PhD
J. Crayton Pruitt Family Department of Biomedical Engineering, University of Florida, Department of Orthopaedic Surgery & Sports Medicine, University of Florida, Gainesville, Florida, USA

LUIGI PIARULLI, MSc
PhD Student, Department of Mechanical Engineering, Drexel University, Philadelphia, Pennsylvania, USA

ROBIN M. QUEEN, PhD
Department of Biomedical Engineering and Mechanics, Kevin P. Granata Biomechanics Lab, Blacksburg, Virginia, USA; Department of Orthopaedic Surgery, Virginia Tech Carilion School of Medicine, Roanoke, Virginia, USA

CHRISTOPHER W. REB, DO
Orthopaedics, Veterans Health Administration North Florida/South Georgia Health System, Malcom Randall VA Medical Center, Gainesville, Florida, USA

DANIEL SCHMITT, PhD
Department of Evolutionary Anthropology, Duke University, Durham, North Carolina, USA

SORIN SIEGLER, PhD
Professor, Department of Mechanical Engineering, Drexel University, Philadelphia, Pennsylvania, USA

PETER A. SMITH, MD
Motion Analysis Center, Shriners Children's Chicago, Chicago, Illinois, USA

JORDAN STOLLE, MSc
PhD Student, Department of Mechanical Engineering, Drexel University, Philadelphia, Pennsylvania, USA

JOHN M. TARAZI, MD
Research Fellow, Donald and Barbara Zucker School of Medicine at Hofstra/Northwell, Hempstead, New York, USA; Department of Orthopaedic Surgery, Northwell Health—Huntington Hospital, Huntington, New York, USA

JASON M. WILKEN, PT, PhD
Department of Physical Therapy and Rehabilitation Science, The University of Iowa, Iowa City, Iowa, USA

Editorial Advisory Board

Contents

Testing with cadaveric foot and ankle specimens began as mechanical techniques to study foot function and then evolved into static simulations of specific instances of gait, before technologies were eventually developed to fully replicate the gait cycle. This article summarizes the clinical applications of dynamic cadaveric gait simulation, including foot bone kinematics and joint function, muscle function, ligament function, orthopaedic foot and ankle pathologies, and total ankle replacements. The literature was reviewed and an in-depth summary was written in each section to highlight one of the more sophisticated simulators. The limitations of dynamic cadaveric simulation were also reviewed.

Advancements in volumetric imaging makes it possible to generate high-resolution three-dimensional reconstructions of bones in throughout the foot and ankle. The use of weightbearing computed tomography allows for the analysis of joint relationships in a consistent natural position that can be used for statistical shape modeling. Using statistical shape modeling, a population-based statistical model is created that can be used to compare mean bone shape morphology and identify anatomical modes of variation. A review is presented to highlight the current work using statistical shape modeling in the foot and ankle with a future view of the impact on clinical care.

This review characterizes fibula mechanics in the context of syndesmosis injury and repair. Through detailed understanding of fibula kinematics (the study of motion) and kinetics (the study of forces that cause motion), the full complexity of fibula motion can be appreciated. Although the magnitudes of fibula rotation and translation are inherently small, even slight alterations of fibula position or movement can substantially impact force propagation through the ankle and hindfoot joints. Accordingly, implications for clinical care are discussed.

Video content accompanies this article at http://www.foot.theclinics. com.

Although not the most prevalent form of lower limb pathology, ankle arthritis is one of the most painful and life-limiting forms of arthritis. Developing from overuse and various traumatic injuries, the effect of ankle arthritis on gait mechanics and effective treatment options for ankle arthritis remain an area of extensive inquiry. Although nonsurgical options are common (physical therapy, limited weight-bearing, and steroidal injections), surgical options are popular with patients. Fusion remains a common approach to stabilize the joint and relieve pain. However, starting in the early 1970s, total ankle arthroplasty was proposed as an alternative to fusion.

FOOT AND ANKLE CLINICS

RELATED SERIES

Orthopedic Clinics
Clinics in Sports Medicine
Physical Medicine and Rehabilitation Clinics

THE CLINICS ARE NOW AVAILABLE ONLINE!
Access your subscription at:
www.theclinics.com

Foreword: Translational Research in Orthopedic Foot and Ankle Surgery

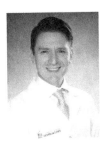

Cesar de Cesar Netto, MD, PhD
Consulting Editor

This issue on "Applied Translational Research in Foot and Ankle Surgery" is definitely a special one. Throughout my career, I have had a unique opportunity to interact and learn with several high-level PhD researchers passionate about orthopedics and foot and ankle surgery. The list is long, and it would be tough to mention all the names here, but Cesar Augusto Martins Pereira in Sao Paulo, Brent Parks and Pooyan Abbasi in Baltimore, and Daniel Sturnick and Howard Hillstrom in New York represent exceptionally well some of the basic science and translational researchers that inspired me to fall in love with foot and ankle and joint biomechanics, for example. After starting at the University of Iowa as an Assistant Professor and Director of the Orthopedic Functional Imaging Research Laboratory, I have then had the honor to have the respected Don Anderson to serve not only as my primary mentor but also as an unbelievable friend and supporter, teaching me a lot in different areas of research and academics. With all that in mind, I thought that an issue on applied translational research in foot and ankle surgery would serve well the *Foot and Ankle Clinics of North America* followers and readers, and Don Anderson was an easy and obvious choice to serve as Guest Editor. He has done an outstanding job, putting together a roster of the most influential translational researchers that focused their careers on the orthopedic foot and ankle. The authors covered different topics, such as ankle instability, gait simulation, alignment, finite-element analysis and shape-modeling, ankle arthritis and total ankle replacement, diabetic foot, syndesmotic injuries, congenital foot and ankle disorders, and more, from a PhD translational research perspective. I'm sure this will be a landmark issue of *Foot and Ankle Clinics of North America* and will serve as a strong reference for researchers and clinicians to consult about translational research in orthopedic foot and ankle surgery.

I hope you all enjoy it.

Foot Ankle Clin N Am 28 (2023) xv–xvi
https://doi.org/10.1016/j.fcl.2023.01.002
1083-7515/23/© 2023 Published by Elsevier Inc.

Have a great, blessed, and healthy 2023!

Cesar de Cesar Netto, MD, PhD
Department of Orthopaedics and Rehabilitation
University of Iowa
200 Hawkins Dr
Iowa City, IA 52242, USA

E-mail address:
cesar-netto@uiowa.edu

Preface

Upping Our Game in Foot and Ankle Research

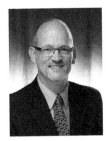

Donald D. Anderson, PhD
Editor

Present-day Orthopedic Foot and Ankle clinical practice is built upon over a century of research, much of that research involving anatomic and cadaveric studies subject to historical limitations that challenge the veracity of its findings. This is not to disrespect those who did the research or the clinical advances it spurred. It is rather simply a statement of cold hard truth. State-of-the-art mechanical testing, biology, imaging, and modeling capabilities have greatly expanded the rigor with which research can be done over the past three decades since I graduated from the University of Iowa with my PhD in mechanical engineering. These new capabilities afford new opportunities to better understand the complex and foundational interplay of biology and mechanics in the foot and ankle, which can lead to evidence-based practice improvements. With an eye admittedly more toward biomechanics (my own specialty), this issue of *Foot and Ankle Clinics of North America* aims to survey some of the latest and greatest work in this context.

It is not a very well-kept secret, but scientists love to measure things. This is because measurement is at its core an objective quantitative process. A quote from Lord Kelvin from the 1880s captures this idea: "When you can measure what you are speaking about, and express it in numbers, you know something about it; but when you cannot measure it, when you cannot express it in numbers, your knowledge is of a meagre and unsatisfactory kind: it may be the beginning of knowledge, but you have scarcely, in your thoughts, advanced to the stage of science, whatever the matter may be."[1] In this vein, the authors contributing to this issue were asked to focus on ways in which new measurement tools and capabilities were being used to address longstanding clinical issues, such as failure of total ankle replacement and the description of complex 3D bony pathologic conditions.

Foot Ankle Clin N Am 28 (2023) xvii–xviii
https://doi.org/10.1016/j.fcl.2022.10.001
1083-7515/23/© 2022 Published by Elsevier Inc.

It has been a pleasure working with such a talented group of scientists to bring this issue to you! Our vision was to query a representative cross-section of the Foot and Ankle Research Community. We focused primarily on PhD researchers who spend most of their time doing rigorous research in this area, without losing sight of its clinical application. It feels as if we are at a critical crossroads in foot and ankle research, with new tools and techniques coming available each year that promise to offer new insights. As representatives of the scientific community, the authors who contributed papers to this issue and I encourage you to join us as we up our game in foot and ankle research.

Donald D. Anderson, PhD
Orthopedic Biomechanics Lab
University of Iowa
200 Newton Road
2181 Westlawn Building
Iowa City, IA 52242, USA

E-mail address:
don-anderson@uiowa.edu

REFERENCES

1. Kelvin WT. Electrical Units of Measurement," a lecture given on 3 May 1883, Published in the Book "Popular Lectures and Addresses, Volume 1: Constitution of Matter, 1891. Macmillan and Company (London). Page, 80.

Biomechanics and Tribology of Total Ankle Replacement

Claire Brockett, PhD

KEYWORDS

• Total ankle replacement • Tribology • Biomechanics

KEY POINTS

- Total ankle replacement has been used since the 1970s but clinical outcomes tend to be less successful than other lower limb joint replacement.
- Range of motion in ankle replacement is typically lower than "normal" control groups but better than ankle fusion and restores function beyond the arthritic ankle.
- Tribology of total ankle replacement has a critical role in clinical survivorship.
- Limited experimental studies to date but demonstrate effect of design and biomechanics on wear performance of a total ankle replacement.
- Retrieval analysis gives insight into biomechanics and tribology of total ankle replacement and indicates adverse loading conditions that are yet to be modeled experimentally.

INTRODUCTION

Osteoarthritis (OA) of the ankle is a degenerative condition, which affects approximately 1% of the adult population.[1] It is frequently associated with previous trauma (severe or recurrent ankle sprain, joint fracture) and typically presents in younger patients than arthritis of the hip or knee. It has a significant impact on patient quality of life.[2] Early-stage interventions may include orthotics and steroidal injections. Surgical interventions, such as total ankle replacement (TAR) and ankle fusion, are often offered as a final option, with ankle fusion still considered the clinical gold standard due to better clinical survivorship. However, recent ankle replacement devices have demonstrated improved performance and offer better biomechanical function compared with ankle fusion, so they are increasing in popularity.[3] This article will give a brief overview of the design development of ankle replacement with specific consideration of biomechanical and tribological performance.

History of Total Ankle Replacement

Total ankle replacement was developed in the 1970s and used the materials and technology that had been applied to total hip and knee replacement in the decades before.

Department of Mechanical Engineering, INSIGNEO Institute for in Silico Medicine, University of Sheffield, UK
E-mail address: CLBrockett@gmail.com

Foot Ankle Clin N Am 28 (2023) 1–12
https://doi.org/10.1016/j.fcl.2022.10.002
1083-7515/23/© 2023 Elsevier Inc. All rights reserved.

Initial approaches did not give full consideration of the natural biomechanics and geometry of the ankle and were often highly constrained or not sufficiently constrained, leading to failure at the fixation interface and damage to the surrounding soft tissues.[4] Often these ankle replacements demonstrated promising initial outcomes but high failure rates were observed beyond 2 years, which led to the intervention being abandoned in clinic for nearly a decade.[5,6]

Second-generation implants sought to address earlier problems by using cementless fixation, which enabled smaller devices and less bone resection than cemented implants, creating semiconstrained, more anatomically representative bearing surfaces and maintaining ligamentous tension.[4] Typically these designs used a 2-component or 3-component implant with metallic tibial and talar components and a polyethylene insert that was either mobile or fixed (**Fig. 1**). Until the last 5 years, a mobile bearing was the more preferred design in Europe because it was considered to give more rotational and translational freedom, aiming to reduce stress at the fixation interface and increasing tolerance to surgical positioning.[7] Conversely, fixed-bearing total ankle replacements have long been the preferred choice in the United States, with the devices considered to provide stability and mitigate risk of polyethylene insert dislocation.[8] These devices showed a significant improvement in clinical outcome but survivorship was still typically around 80% at 10 years post implant, much lower than the successful outcomes of hip or knee replacement.[4]

In addition to the design of the bearing surface, there continues to exist a wide variety of fixation features across different total ankle replacements ranging from long tibial stems, screw fixation, and smaller bars/lugs. Each of these has different proposed benefits including improved stability, early fixation, and more physiologic stress distribution to the bone but also have concerns including stress shielding, implant loosening, and elevated contact stress due to reduced contact area, respectively, so an optimized fixation solution seems to not yet be achieved.[9]

More recent designs have reflected improvements in materials technology, such as the use of cross-linked polyethylene,[10] as well as advances in surgical instrumentation to improve implant positioning and soft tissue balancing.[11] These devices are currently quite early in their clinical use, so literature is typically outlining short-term to medium-term performance (up to 5 years), which often also includes surgeon learning-curves[12] but the overall picture for these new devices is promising.

Clinical failure in total ankle replacement (requiring revision surgery) is often associated with aseptic loosening and osteolysis[13–15]—with osteolytic lesions considered to be associated with strain within the bone, stress shielding, and immune response to wear debris[16]—hence, the biomechanics and biotribology of ankle replacements are important factors in clinical outcome and patient satisfaction.

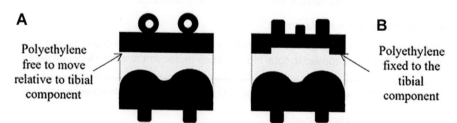

Fig. 1. A mobile-bearing (*A*) and fixed-bearing (*B*) total ankle replacements—nominally based on MatOrtho BOX and Wright Medical Infinity designs, respectively (current generation devices).[8] (Image courtesy of Dr Alexandra Smyth.)

CURRENT EVIDENCE: BIOMECHANICS

To consider the biomechanics of total ankle replacement, we first need to consider the joints the device replaces and their contribution to overall motion at the ankle. In a total ankle replacement, metallic bearing components are fixed to the tibia and talus, with the polyethylene insert located between these 2 bearings (**Fig. 2**[17]). Several cointerventions, including fixation of the syndesmosis or sub-talar fusion,[18] have been adopted during TAR surgery; however, compared with primary total ankle replacement, the incidence of cointervention is rare.

Motion of the whole ankle complex occurs primarily in the sagittal plane, with dorsi/plantar-flexion contributing a maximum range of motion of 65° to 75°, most of which occurs at the talocrural joint.[19] Rotation and inversion-eversion are considered to occur at both the talocrural and sub-talar joints, although the sub-talar joint contributes more to the overall range of motion. Conventional gait analysis enables us to quantify the motion of the overall ankle joint complex but is unable to separate the motions of the sub-talar and talocrural joints. Hence, the biomechanical data presented in this article will largely explore whole joint function of different ankle replacements.

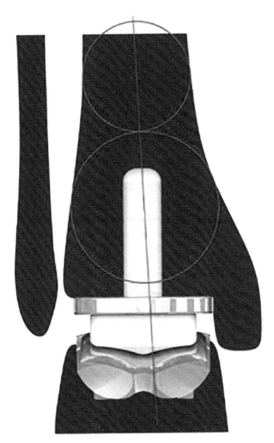

Coronal

Fig. 2. Exemplar of a total ankle replacement with tibial axis indicated.[17] (Image by Ashley Stratton-Powell, licenced under CC BY-NC-SA 2.5)

One of design requirements of total ankle replacement is the preservation of range of motion, compared with ankle arthrodesis. Early biomechanical studies of first-generation total ankle replacements tended to indicate no improvement in range of motion or cadence postoperatively, although this may well be related to the challenges of those early devices.[4,19]

Studies exploring second-generation and third-generation ankle replacements have tended to compare devices against the alternative clinical treatment—ankle arthrodesis—and typically demonstrate improved range of motion, particularly within the sagittal plane for the TAR cohorts.[20,21] Biomechanical studies suggest that patients with TAR are able to perform daily activities more efficiently than patients with fusion. Increased plantarflexion and higher ankle power in TAR cohorts indicates a better ability to propel the foot forward.[22] Conversely, ankle fusion—due to the rigidity of the ankle joint complex—exhibits an increased moment arm through the foot, meaning dorsiflexion moments are distributed across other joints of the foot, which may contribute to the adjacent joint arthritis that is sometimes observed.[23]

Many of the gait studies and models of the ankle use rigid single-segment foot models, which do not isolate the true motion of the tibiotalar joint and therefore also include any compensatory mechanisms of adjacent joints. Additionally, clinical biomechanics studies rely on skin markers to derive motion of bones that are not adjacent to the skin—it is simply not possible to mount a marker on the skin over the talus. Therefore, we rely on multisegment models to model the predicted behavior of the talus, based on the motion of other joints in the foot and lower limb. Few multisegment models have been published for total ankle replacement but they indicate higher range of motion in the rearfoot and forefoot in ankle replacement compared with fusion but significantly lower range of motion than the control group.[24–26] Overall, it seems that TAR does have the capacity to improve range of motion compared with ankle fusion and, in some cases, has been shown to surpass preoperative range of motion of the arthritic ankle but it does not seem to fully restore function comparable to a "normal" ankle.

Most recently, fluoroscopic studies have been introduced that use imaging to visualize and measure the motion at the talocrural joint. This method gives us the most accurate information regarding biomechanical function of the ankle replacement. Comparison between the implanted ankle and the contralateral limb or control subjects indicated minor reductions in range of motion (particularly dorsiflexion) compared with control subjects but this was relatively small.[27]

Clinical Relevance: Biomechanics

Improved and more natural range of motion is often cited as a potential benefit of total ankle replacement when compared with ankle fusion for the treatment of end-stage ankle OA. Studies have shown that typically the range of motion is better with replacement but it does not achieve the full range of motion of a "healthy" ankle joint. This may be related to features other than the ankle replacement itself, including soft tissue tension and the function before surgery. As an end-stage treatment, patients often wait a substantial time period before undergoing surgery, and changes to limb function during this period may impair the potential to recover full joint function. Prehab and postoperative physiotherapy is variable, and there is considerable scope for optimizing rehabilitation to improve biomechanical outcomes.

The improved range of motion of the talocrural joint compared with fusion, and lack of compensation at the sub-talar joint, does suggest that the better biomechanical function prevents the localized joint degeneration of the mid-foot and sub-talar joint sometimes characterized in failure of ankle fusion.

Current Evidence: Tribology

Tribology can be defined as the science of 2 interacting surfaces in relative motion and specifically refers to the friction, wear, and lubrication of the articulation. In total ankle replacement, tribological related failure (wear and implant breakage), accounts for approximately 13% to 17% of all failures, with a further 19% to 38% of failure associated with aseptic loosening, which may also be linked to implant wear.[13]

Although experimental friction studies have been conducted in the hip and knee, for natural and replacement joints, very limited research has been undertaken for total ankle replacement. Wear testing of total ankle replacement is also limited (<10 studies published as full journal articles) when compared with hip and knee replacement, largely due to total ankle replacement being classified as Class II devices until recently, thereby previously not requiring the same level of in vitro testing before market approval. Indeed, although there has been an international standard (ISO standard) for wear testing of hip replacements for more than 2 decades (ISO 14242–1), the ISO standard for wear testing of total ankle replacements[28] (ISO22622–2019) has been introduced only in the last few years, and as yet, there are no published studies using this standard.

The 3 most-commonly observed wear mechanisms in total joint replacement are adhesion, abrasion, and fatigue. Adhesion and abrasion often occur together and contribute most to the generation of particulate wear debris in joint replacement in a normally functioning implant. Fatigue is associated with the high cyclic loads the materials undergo through every day activities and depends on the implant geometry and patient biomechanics. Experimental wear simulation typically tests an implant at a rate of 1 Hz (approximate walking speed) for several million cycles (proposed to be equivalent to 5 or more years of in vivo activity) under loading and motion conditions representative of the gait cycle—meaning that wear mechanisms in these studies are mostly adhesion and abrasion.

All ankle replacement wear tests conducted to date use an adapted knee wear simulator, such that the implant is tested in an inverted position.[29–34] It is therefore important to consider the axes of motion of the simulator with regards to the in vivo ankle biomechanics when conducting the tests to ensure the conditions are clinically representative (**Fig. 3**).[35] Wear testing has been conducted in several studies using a range of kinematic inputs, derived from clinical biomechanics data, based on healthy subjects. There is some discussion regarding whether ankle wear simulation should be conducted using inputs derived from total ankle replacement subjects but as discussed earlier, the range of motion and potentially the loading are often reduced compared with "normal" healthy subjects, and therefore testing with "normal" gait inputs is considered a more demanding test condition.

The published studies cover a range of devices, materials, and bearing designs and, although limited in number, do provide a good overview of performance of ankle joint replacement. The biomechanical inputs used vary slightly between authors, with plantar-dorsiflexion generally totally approximately 30° of motion. Similarly, total rotation is approximately 10° across almost all studies (specific ROM is shown in **Table 1**). Most studies have also conducted their simulation under displacement control, where the simulator drives the motions by a specified displacement. One study has used force-controlled inputs, derived from studies on cadaveric specimens—force-controlled simulation is thought to more closely model the soft tissue behavior but the local displacements of the bearing are not controlled and therefore the motion may be more variable.[33] Notably most of these simulations do not have any inputs for version—this may be due to the capacity of the simulator or the presumption that version occurs at the sub-talar joint.

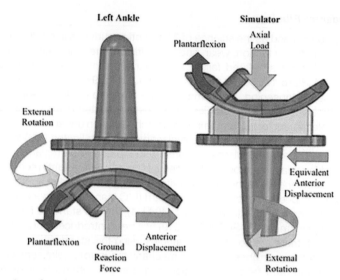

Fig. 3. Direction of motion in wear-simulation versus in vivo motion. (Image courtesy of Dr Alexandra Smyth.)

Axial load, however, varies significantly between studies. Based on the dynamic force profile presented by Stauffer and colleagues, most studies approximated a peak load of 5 times body weight. However, both Reinders and colleagues[33] and Affatato and colleagues[30] used a load of approximately half this—around 1.6 kN. It is important to attempt to represent the in vivo condition as closely as possible, and therefore, it is critical to consider the clinical biomechanics in developing such test methodologies.

In addition to small variations between kinematics, the number of cycles tested and, in some cases, the lubricant used in the test are also varied. In most studies, bovine calf serum was used—specified either as a concentration (eg, Bell and Fisher[29] used 25% calf serum supplemented with 0.1% sodium azide) or as a required protein concentration of 20 g/L—which is representative of the ISO standard requirements for lubrication media in testing of total knee replacement. Affatato *and colleagues* highlighted their lubrication choice of deionized water as a limitation of their study because it is known to be poor at representing the in vivo lubrication and hence effects the wear rate.[30]

Table 1				
Ranges of motion in TAR wear studies				
Author	Plantar-Flexion	Dorsi-Flexion	Internal Rotation	External Rotation
Bell,[29] 2007	15°	15°	2°	8°
Affatato et al,[30] 2007	20°	10°	2.6°	7.7°
Postak 2008	20°	10°	2°	2°
Bischoff et al,[32] 2015	16°	15.2°	2°	8°
Reinders et al,[33] 2015	5°	10°	0°	10°
Smyth et al,[31] 2017	15°	15°	2.3°	8°
ISO 22622[28] 2019	15°	15°	2°	8°

The influence of simulator has been well noted in other joint replacement wear studies, meaning comparison between studies needs to be cautious. However, we can see across most studies that wear rates have been quite similar. Smyth and colleagues demonstrated that while there was a significant change in wear when contrasting unidirectional and multidirectional inputs (no rotation/no AP v. rotation/AP), the magnitude of anterior-posterior (AP) displacement had no influence on wear rate.[31] Previously, it had been recognized in fixed-bearing knee replacement that the kinematic inputs had a significant influence on wear performance due to the behavior of polyethylene.[36] When motion is applied in one direction, the polyethylene chains align and undergo strain hardening, which improves wear resistance in that direction. Conversely, multidirectional motion causes the chain orientation to continually change resulting in shearing of polyethylene from the surface, generating elevated wear. Rotating platform knee replacements demonstrate (in the laboratory) lower wear rates than fixed-bearing knees under multidirectional motion because there is a decoupling of motion, such that flexion and displacement (unidirectional motion) occurs on the superior surface of the insert, and rotation (another unidirectional motion) occurs on the inferior surface. This effectively creates 2 unidirectional (low) wear articulations. However, Smyth and colleagues demonstrated that the equivalent benefit was not achieved in a mobile-bearing total ankle replacement—with AP displacement and rotation occurring at the tibial interface, and the primary flexion motion occurring at the more conforming talar interface—and this is perhaps reflected across all the mobile-bearing TAR wear data to date.[31] The only fixed-bearing total ankle replacement with published wear data is the Zimmer Trabecular Metal with conventional and cross-linked polyethylene.[32] This showed a lower wear rate than any of the mobile-bearing ankle replacements, and this may be related to the bearing design. As previously observed with other joint replacements, the introduction of a cross-linked polyethylene has a significant influence on wear rates (**Table 2**).

Another method that helps us understand the tribology of total ankle replacement is retrieval analysis. To date, there has been limited published research in the area but the findings so far do indicate some key factors to consider and enable us to more closely link the biomechanics and tribological performance.[17,37,38]

These retrieval analyses have covered a range of ankle replacement designs, including mobile and fixed-bearing TARs, and while the wear studies have highlighted that fixed-bearing TARs may have better wear performance, the limited retrieval studies have suggested that mobile-bearing TARs are a lower risk for loosening.[37] Surface damage, scratching and pitting were observed on all polyethylene bearings—with fixed-bearing devices typically showing more damage to the posterior aspect of the insert than the anterior aspect—and it has been proposed that this may indicate constraint during gait that is either related to device or surgical technique, with elevated stress posteriorly contributing to early failure of the devices.[38] Mobile-bearing ankle replacements have more frequently demonstrated edge-loading and impingement, suggesting that they could be vulnerable to insert migration.[17,37] Furthermore, polyethylene transfer has been observed on the tibial component reflecting the shape of the insert—suggesting that the ankle replacement does not experience much relative motion in vivo (**Fig. 4**) compared with wear simulation—and this may be related to the tension within the joint and the restraint of the soft tissues that are not modeled in vitro. Failure associated with insert fracture indicates elevated contact stress within the ankle joint.[39] The ankle joint is relatively small, and experiences loads of up to 5 times body weight during walking. Several studies have explored the contact mechanics in ankle replacement[40] and have demonstrated that contact pressure can be close to the yield strength of polyethylene, even when

Table 2
Reported wear rates for TAR

Author	Implant	Samples	Cycles (Million)	Wear Rate (mm³/MC)
Bell,[29] 2007 (No AP)	BP	3	5	10.4 ± 11.8
	Mobility	3	5	3.4 ± 10.0
(With AP)	BP	3	1	16.4 ± 17.4
	Mobility	3	1	10.4 ± 14.7
Affatato et al,[30] 2007	BOX	3	2	18.6 ± 12.8
Postak 2008	STAR	5	10	5.7 ± 2.1
Bischoff et al,[32] 2015	Trabecular Metal (CPE)	3	5	8.0 ± 1.4
	Trabecular Metal (XPE)	3	5	2.1 ± 0.3
Reinders et al,[33] 2015	Hintegra	3	3	18.2 ± 1.4
Smyth et al,[31] 2017 (4 mm AP)	Zenith	5	2	13.3 ± 2.5
(9 mm AP)	Zenith	5	2	11.8 ± 3.7
Hopwood 2019 (Medium)	BOX	6	5	11.00 ± 3.06
(XS)	BOX	6	5	10.64 ± 4.61

well aligned, so it is not unreasonable to assume that an adverse loading event, either through altered biomechanics or poor implant alignment,[41] could cause elevated stress that would result in insert breakage, and this is likely to be through sustained loading and caused by fatigue, resulting in cracking of the polyethylene.

Clinical Relevance: Tribology

Approximately 50% of clinical failure of total ankle replacement may be associated with tribological causes wear, implant breakage, and loosening, so understanding and improving performance is critical to TAR longevity. Experimental wear studies indicate the benefits of a mobile-bearing seen within total knee replacement are not translated to improved TAR wear performance due to differences in how the implant functions. However, limited retrieval analysis also indicates that mobile-bearing TARs may be less susceptible to early loosening, so there is currently a mixed picture in determining optimal implant design. Experimental wear rates seem to be similar to total knee replacement, and therefore, it may be expected that wear-mediated osteolysis could become a clinical issue. The use of a cross-linked polyethylene insert could mitigate the wear rate but the trade-off in cross-linking with mechanical properties may become of concern for an insert that is so thin—indeed, fracture of inserts tends to be observed where thickness is 4 mm or lower.[38]

- Limited, but increasing, wear studies for total ankle replacement.
- Fixed-bearing TAR has lowest wear rate of all studies but retrieval analysis suggests higher risk of loosening, so there is no definitive design for optimal TAR performance to date.

DISCUSSION

Total ankle replacement has the potential to provide an end-stage intervention for ankle arthritis while improving the quality of life and partially restoring joint biomechanics. Compared with fusion, ankle replacement offers more natural function and seems less affected by adjacent joint arthritis; however, clinical outcomes are still less satisfactory than other lower limb joint replacements with a failure rate of 10% or more after 10 years.

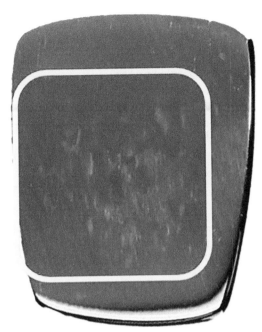

Fig. 4. Example of polyethylene transfer imprint of bearing insert.

Clinical failure mechanisms include implant breakage and wear, and therefore, the tribology of a device is critical to the success. Failure such as insert fracture suggests the stresses within the joint have exceeded the mechanical properties of the implant and, therefore, material selection and implant design should be optimized to yield the best combination of good mechanical properties and low contact stress. However, the design does not function in isolation, use of surgical technique and instrumentation that enables consistent and predictable implant placement is important in reducing the risk of adverse loading conditions.

The interplay between biomechanics and tribology needs further consideration about the implant design. No experimental wear study to date has included inversion/eversion as a simulator input, and yet we know that in a natural, healthy ankle, some degree of version can occur at the talocrural joint. The most recent fluoroscopy study demonstrated small amounts of version occurring in the total joint replacement, although less than healthy controls, and it highlights the need to consider whether the devices are designed to tolerate these motions. For example, if a mobile-bearing design with a flat/flat tibial interface and a highly conforming talar interface were to experience version moments, would the inherent constraint of the device resist this motion, resulting in elevated stress within the joint—or would the mobile nature of the insert enable motion to occur? These are factors we do not yet understand and could be key in unlocking longer term clinical success.

Development in both biomechanical analysis and tribological simulation within the last decade have enabled us to understand many aspects of ankle replacement function and will enable us to further advance total ankle replacement design with a goal of improving biomechanical function, patient quality of life, and clinical outcome.

CLINICS CARE POINTS

- Biomechanical function of patients with TAR is better than with fusion and demonstrates improvement on biomechanics of arthritic ankles.
- Rehabilitation therapies have been underreported in ankle literature and could be key to improving functional outcome of TAR.
- Difference in biomechanics between ankle replacement and fusion reflect associated failures relating to adjacent joint arthritis and degeneration in ankle fusion.
- Wear of total ankle replacement depends on several factors including surgical positioning and implant alignment.

DISCLOSURE

The author has received financial and in-kind research support from Corin Group, United Kingdom and MatOrtho Ltd, in addition to institutional support from EPSRC, United Kingdom and NIHR, United Kingdom.

REFERENCES

1. Saltzman CL, Salamon ML, Blanchard GM, et al. Epidemiology of ankle arthritis: report of a consecutive series of 639 patients from a tertiary orthopaedic center. Iowa orthopaedic J 2005;25:44.
2. Glazebrook M, Daniels T, Younger A, et al. Comparison of health-related quality of life between patients with end-stage ankle and hip arthrosis. JBJS 2008;90(3): 499–505.
3. Terrell RD, Montgomery SR, Pannell WC, et al. Comparison of practice patterns in total ankle replacement and ankle fusion in the United States. Foot Ankle Int 2013; 34(11):1486–92.
4. Vickerstaff JA, Miles AW, Cunningham JL. A brief history of total ankle replacement and a review of the current status. Med Eng Phys 2007;29(10):1056–64.
5. Lord G, Marotte JH. Total ankle replacement (author's transl). Revue de chirurgie orthopedique et reparatrice de l'appareil moteur 1980;66(8):527–30.
6. Gougoulias NE, Khanna A, Maffulli N. History and evolution in total ankle arthroplasty. Br Med Bull 2009;89(1):111–51.
7. Cifaldi AJ, Barton EC, Roukis TS, et al. Total ankle replacement based on worldwide registry data trends. InPrimary and revision total ankle replacement 2021 (pp. 13-27). Springer, Cham.
8. Kooner S, Marsh A, Wilson IR, et al. History of total ankle replacement in north America. InPrimary and revision total ankle replacement. Cham: Springer; 2021. p. 3–12.
9. Sopher RS, Amis AA, Calder JD, et al. Total ankle replacement design and positioning affect implant-bone micromotion and bone strains. Med Eng Phys 2017; 42:80–90.
10. Schipper ON, Haddad SL, Fullam S, et al. Wear characteristics of conventional ultrahigh-molecular-weight polyethylene versus highly cross-linked polyethylene in total ankle arthroplasty. Foot Ankle Int 2018;39(11):1335–44.
11. Choi WJ, Kim BS, Lee JW. Preoperative planning and surgical technique: how do I balance my ankle? Foot Ankle Int 2012;33(3):244–9.
12. Simonson DC, Roukis TS. Incidence of complications during the surgeon learning curve period for primary total ankle replacement: a systematic review. Clin Podiatric Med Surg 2015;32(4):473–82.

13. NJR for England, Wales N. Ireland and the Isle of Man 2021. National Joint Registry 18th Annual Report. National Joint Registry | 18th Annual Report. [Online]. Available from: www.njrcentre.org.uk. Accessed 5 May 2022.
14. Zaidi R, Cro S, Gurusamy K, et al. The outcome of total ankle replacement: a systematic review and meta-analysis. Bone Joint J 2013;95(11):1500–7.
15. Espinosa N, Wirth SH. Revision of the aseptic and septic total ankle replacement. Clin Podiatric Med Surg 2013;30(2):171–85.
16. Besse JL. Osteolytic cysts with total ankle replacement: frequency and causes? Foot Ankle Surg official J Eur Soc Foot Ankle Surgeons 2015;21(2):75–6.
17. Stratton-Powell AA. On the failure of total ankle replacement: a retrieval analysis PhD Thesis, University of Leeds. https://etheses.whiterose.ac.uk/20588/. [Accessed 19 April 2022].
18. Usuelli FG, Maccario C, Manzi L, et al. Clinical outcome and fusion rate following simultaneous subtalar fusion and total ankle arthroplasty. Foot Ankle Int 2016; 37(7):696–702.
19. Stauffer RN, Chao EY, Brewster RC. Force and motion analysis of the normal, diseased, and prosthetic ankle joint. Clin orthopaedics Relat Res 1977;(127): 189–96.
20. Segal AD, Cyr KM, Stender CJ, et al. A three-year prospective comparative gait study between patients with ankle arthrodesis and arthroplasty. Clin Biomech 2018;54:42–53.
21. Ingrosso S, Benedetti MG, Leardini A, et al. GAIT analysis in patients operated with a novel total ankle prosthesis. Gait & posture 2009;30(2):132–7.
22. Hahn ME, Wright ES, Segal AD, et al. Comparative gait analysis of ankle arthrodesis and arthroplasty: initial findings of a prospective study. Foot Ankle Int 2012; 33(4):282–9.
23. Ling JS, Smyth NA, Fraser EJ, et al. Investigating the relationship between ankle arthrodesis and adjacent-joint arthritis in the hindfoot: a systematic review. JBJS 2015;97(6):513–9.
24. Fritz JM, Canseco K, Konop KA, et al. Multi-segment foot kinematics during gait following ankle arthroplasty. J Orthopaedic Research®. 2022;40(3):685–94.
25. Seo SG, Kim EJ, Lee DJ, et al. Comparison of multisegmental foot and ankle motion between total ankle replacement and ankle arthrodesis in adults. Foot Ankle Int 2017;38(9):1035–44.
26. Sanders AE, Kraszewski AP, Ellis SJ, et al. Differences in gait and stair ascent after total ankle arthroplasty and ankle arthrodesis. Foot Ankle Int 2021;42(3): 347–55.
27. Lenz AL, Lisonbee RJ, Peterson AC, et al. Total ankle replacement provides symmetrical postoperative kinematics: a biplane fluoroscopy imaging study. Foot Ankle Int 2022;43(6):818–29.
28. ISO 22622:2019(en) Implants for surgery — Wear of total ankle-joint prostheses — Loading and displacement parameters for wear-testing machines with load or displacement control and corresponding environmental conditions for test.
29. Bell CJ, Fisher J. Simulation of polyethylene wear in ankle joint prostheses. J Biomed Mater Res B: Appl Biomater 2007;81(1):162–7. The Japanese Society for Biomaterials, and The Australian Society for Biomaterials and the Korean Society for Biomaterials.
30. Affatato S, Leardini A, Leardini W, et al. Meniscal wear at a three-component total ankle prosthesis by a knee joint simulator. J Biomech 2007;40(8):1871–6.
31. Smyth A, Fisher J, Suñer S, et al. Influence of kinematics on the wear of a total ankle replacement. J Biomech 2017;53:105–10.

32. Bischoff JE, Fryman JC, Parcell J, et al. Influence of crosslinking on the wear performance of polyethylene within total ankle arthroplasty. Foot Ankle Int 2015; 36(4):369–76.
33. Reinders J, von Stillfried F, Altan E, et al. Force-controlled dynamic wear testing of total ankle replacements. Acta Biomater 2015;12:332–40.
34. Hopwood J, Redmond A, Chapman G, et al. Influence of implant size on the wear performance of a total ankle arthroplasty. InOrthopaedic Proc 2020;102(1):64. The British Editorial Society of Bone & Joint Surgery.
35. Smyth A., Wear of a Total Ankle Replacement PhD thesis, University of Leeds, Available at: https://etheses.whiterose.ac.uk/19367/.
36. McEwen HM, Barnett PI, Bell CJ, et al. The influence of design, materials and kinematics on the in vitro wear of total knee replacements. J Biomech 2005;38(2): 357–65.
37. Currier BH, Hecht PJ, Nunley JA, et al. Analysis of failed ankle arthroplasty components. Foot Ankle Int 2019;40(2):131–8.
38. Ho NC, Park SH, Campbell P, et al. Damage patterns in polyethylene fixed bearings of retrieved total ankle replacements. Foot Ankle Surg 2021;27(3):316–20.
39. Koivu H, Kohonen I, Mattila K, et al. Long-term results of scandinavian total ankle replacement. Foot Ankle Int 2017;38(7):723–31.
40. Terrier A, Larrea X, Guerdat J, et al. Development and experimental validation of a finite element model of total ankle replacement. J Biomech 2014;47(3):742–5.
41. van Hoogstraten SW, Hermus J, Loenen AC, et al. Malalignment of the total ankle replacement increases peak contact stresses on the bone-implant interface: a finite element analysis. BMC Musculoskelet Disord 2022;23(1):1–9.

Diabetic Foot Considerations Related to Plantar Pressures and Shear

Jessi K. Martin, BS, Brian L. Davis, PhD*

KEYWORDS

- Diabetes • Shear and pressure • Instrumentation • Skin ulceration
- Charcot neuroarthropathy

KEY POINTS

- Diabetic foot ulcers are one of the most common complications of diabetes mellitus, with 15% to 25% of these individuals developing a foot ulcer within their lifetime.
- In the presence of neuropathy, there is convincing evidence linking high pressures to the development of diabetic foot ulcers. However, the location of skin breakdown does not correlate well with sites of elevated pressure.
- Given the weak correlation between peak pressure and ulcer location, it is believed that some form of shear (possibly coupled with pressure), is likely to contribute to ulceration.
- Measurement of shear or frictional forces is not routine clinical practice, due to technical issues, the infancy of research in this area, and challenges associated with physical interfaces that are affected by moisture, weave patterns, and sock stiffness.

CLINICAL SIGNIFICANCE OF DIABETIC FOOT ULCERATION

Diabetic foot ulcers (DFUs) are one of the most common complications to diabetes mellitus. Globally, the annual incidence of DFUs is 9.1 to 26.1 million, with 15% to 25% of people with diabetes developing a foot ulcer within their lifetime.[1] The most common complication of foot ulceration is infection/and or amputation, with over 50% of ulcers becoming infectious.[1,2] Once the ulcer has formed, approximately 20% of moderate to severe ulcer cases require amputation.[2] In assessing the mortality rates for foot ulceration and diabetes-related foot amputations, after 5 years the mortality rate of DFU is about 30% and increases to about 50% to 70% after amputation.[2,3] A compounding issue for the clinician is the reoccurrence of DFU once they've healed. Within 1-year post healing, patients have a 40% risk of DFU reoccurrence. This risk increases to 60% within 3 years and 65% within 5 years.[4] The factors

Center for Human Machine Systems, Cleveland State University, WH 305, Cleveland, OH 44115, USA
* Corresponding author.
E-mail address: B.L.Davis@csuohio.edu

Foot Ankle Clin N Am 28 (2023) 13–25
https://doi.org/10.1016/j.fcl.2022.11.004
1083-7515/23/© 2022 Elsevier Inc. All rights reserved.

that increase the risk of ulcer reoccurrence include but are not limited to: a hemoglobin A1C value above 7.5, presence of osteomyelitis, and a geriatric depression scale score greater than or equal to 10 (**Fig. 1**).[2]

As evidenced by the statistics above, DFU is a significant issue in health care settings as well as to patient well-being and clinical outcomes. The etiology of DFU is multifaceted (see **Fig. 1**) and stems from prolonged periods of poor glycemic control (**Fig. 2**).[5–9] It has been well documented that poor glycemic control results in the disruption and dysregulation of the motor, sensory, and autonomic nervous systems resulting in peripheral neuropathy as well as cardiovascular disruptions.[2,10,11] Peripheral Arterial and/or Vascular Disease (PAD and PVD) are compounding risk factors that aid in the development of DFUs. Approximately 10% to 20% of people with diabetes will develop peripheral arterial disease.[12] PAD causes damage to blood vessels including, atherosclerotic blockages, increased thickness of capillary basement membranes, and arteriolar wall hardening.[13] This vessel damage restricts the blood flow through vessels, which decreases overall circulation through body tissues.

Peripheral neuropathy has been shown to disrupt normal gait, causing unsteadiness, gait abnormalities, and pressure distribution changes.[10,14–18] In addition to gait disturbances, peripheral neuropathy also impacts the skin integrity. These disruptions include increased skin dryness, which increases the likelihood of skin breakage, decreased skin integrity as a whole, and decreased muscle-tone which alters the surface area of the foot and disrupts normal load distributions.[13]

There has been a well-established relationship between high-pressure distributions under the foot (greater than 6 kg/cm^2 or 588.4 kPa) and the development of DFUs.[19,20] Periods of high pressure or prolonged applied pressure damage the tissues on and under the applied pressure as they do not allow blood vessels to replenish the nutrients to maintain healthy tissue. In addition, the decreased circulation from neuropathy and diabetes will further restrict the body's ability to replenish required nutrients. This creates further damage through tissue ischemia and results in pressure ulcers that will

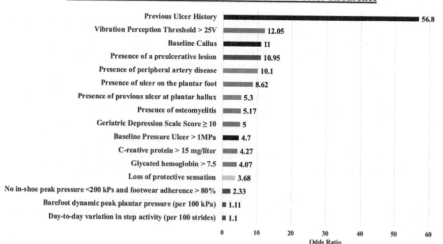

Fig. 1. DFU risk factors independently associated with ulcer recurrence from five different studies. Results from Dubský and colleagues,[5] Reiber and colleagues,[6] Monami and colleagues,[7] Waaijam and colleagues,[8] and Peters and colleagues,[9] and Murray and colleagues[10] are illustrated in blue, yellow, green, burnt orange, pink, and purple, respectively.

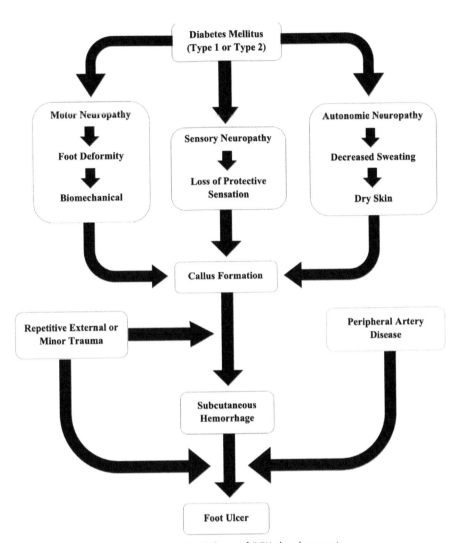

Fig. 2. Flow diagram of the common etiology of DFU development.

not heal.[21] In fact, peripheral ischemia in branching blood vessels leads to ulceration at a case rate of 35%.[13]

However, areas of high pressure are not always indicative of pressure ulcer development in the feet. In fact, only 30% of ulcer locations correlate with peak pressure areas under the foot.[22] Shear is another biomechanical parameter that has assisted in identifying the cause of DFU in areas of the foot. Shear significantly decreases the required applied pressure to cause tissue ischemia.[21] In physics, there is rarely a case where there is an applied pressure force and not some sort of applied shear force (**Fig. 3**).

Current clinical guidelines for DFU treatment include wound debridement, dressings, off-loading and glycemic control.[23] However, these treatments are successful when the foot is offloaded sufficiently, and the ulcer diagnosed early. When using pressure measurements to assist in the assessment of the correct offloading footwear,

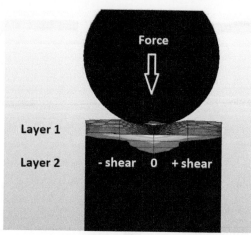

Fig. 3. Simple physics model illustrating shear is zero where pressure is highest, shear stresses have opposite signs on either side of highest pressure, and discontinuity between dermal layers.

the offloading capacity of the footwear is increased and the risk for re-ulceration decreases by 46% to 65%.[24] Bus *and colleagues* showed that when footwear treatment for DFU is designed according to pressure measurements (in this case decreasing the peak pressure experienced in the foot by 20%), patients saw a decrease in the rate of ulcer reoccurrence when compared with treatments not specifically designed through pressure measurement.[25] The caveat here is that patients must adhere to the prescribed wear time of the footwear. Similarly, Ulbrecht *and colleagues* showed that treatment orthoses developed based on foot shape and barefoot plantar pressure, decrease the reoccurrence rate of DFUs.[26]

SHEAR VERSUS PRESSURE

Pressure and shear measurements undoubtedly play an important role in the prevention of DFUs (see **Fig. 3**). From a simplistic standpoint, pressure patterns under the foot are considerably easier to measure and interpret. Both patients and clinicians can appreciate the concept of high plantar pressure. Interpretations of shear, or frictional forces are considerably more challenging. For example, it may be common to think that pressure and shear are simply related by the coefficient of friction, yet, for patients stepping on a pressure platform, pressure and shear are almost never related to each other.[27] In fact, shear can often be zero at the point where pressure is highest (see **Fig. 3**). Visualizing pressure may be straightforward (**Fig. 4**A). However, trying to determine what leads to a particular shear pattern (**Fig. 4**B) requires combining influences of foot twisting, sliding and frictional differences across multiple sensors. Finally, shear can occur in multiple planes, including the sagittal and frontal planes. The current focus is on plantar pressure and shear. It is possible that downward movement of metatarsal heads relative to tissue interspersed between these structures could lead to vertical shearing that in turn could attenuate blood supply to vulnerable tissues (**Fig. 5**).

Although the emphasis has generally been on the magnitudes and locations of peak stresses, the *ratio* of pressures and shear magnitudes is also altered in patients with diabetic neuropathy. This may be indicative of future ulcer development.[28,29] In

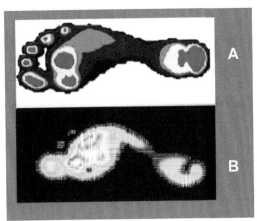

Fig. 4. (*A*): Peak pressure recordings under a patients foot. (*B*): Shear stress distribution. Note that shear can be zero (*black regions*) where pressure may be high, and shearing under the heel does not resemble pressure mapping.

considering shear on the plantar surface of the foot, Davis[30] referred to the "wrinkled carpet effect". Although simplistic, the concept illustrates the challenge of combining shear and pressure data. Pressure values can be considered alone—as evidenced by hundreds of publications on pressure thresholds, locations, and integrals over the gait

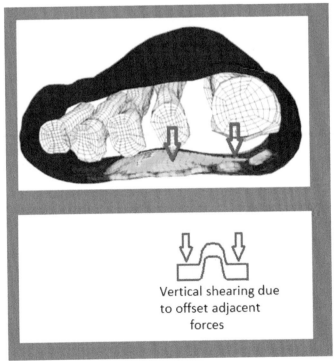

Vertical shearing due to offset adjacent forces

Fig. 5. Shear can occur in multiple planes besides acting on the plantarsurface of the foot. The illustration above shows the concept of vertical shear, caused by adjacent bony structures moving relative to interspersed tissue.

cycle. All that is needed are pressure values at each location under the foot. These data lead to the common graphic (see **Fig. 2**A) depicting "hills and valleys" of pressure information. When shear data are included, the situation becomes more complicated, much like the scenario that leads to a wrinkled carpet! In this case, it is not only pressure that needs to be considered, but also shear, *at locations other than where pressure is being monitored*. A carpet becomes wrinkled when there is a combination of high pressure (due to the leg of a table) and some horizontal force at a different location that causes a portion of the carpet to slide. Naturally, there are multiple places where horizontal forces can be high, which means that for 100 pressure measurements, with each one being paired with shear measurements in anterior, posterior, medial and lateral directions, 400 shear/pressure ratios may need to be analyzed. If one then adds the possibility that a foot is twisting about a vertical axis during stance, then the options for determining risk of skin damage increase even further. To the authors' knowledge, there have not been any studies examining these combinatorial loading scenarios and ulcer risk.

HISTORY OF THE PLANTAR PRESSURE AND SHEAR MEASUREMENTS AS RELATED TO ULCERS

Given the weak correlation between peak pressure and ulcer location,[10,31] it is believed that some form of shear (possibly coupled with pressure), is likely to contribute to ulceration.[32–34] Before 2000, few researchers investigated skin shearing due to the difficulty in constructing devices capable of measuring frictional forces.[35–37] Most devices were uni-directional, leading to underestimates of true shearing stresses.[38–42] In the early 1990's, Lord and colleagues[43] developed a bi-directional sensor that could be placed in an inlay to permit in-shoe measurement. One limitation of this form of discrete sensor is that prior knowledge is required about the areas of interest to determine its placement (eg, under a metatarsal head). As a result, areas experiencing high stresses may remain undetected if they do not coincide with the areas of interest determined *a priori*.

In addition, in the 1990's, Huo and Nicol[44] reported on the development of a three-dimensional force distribution measurement system using strain gauge technology. The device consisted of an array of 336 sensors. Although no pressure or shear data were described, the authors reported that the device was suitable for investigating foot loading conditions during the takeoff phase of the high jump.

Over 20 years ago, leaders in diabetic foot research[45] commented "the measurement of shear stress continues to be an elusive goal". Not much has changed since that time! For the past 30 years, numerous companies have entered the market with new technologies related to pressure (most commonly) or shear (rarely). In general, the devices on the market are for assessing overground pressure profiles or, less commonly, in-shoe stresses. There are currently no companies selling in-shoe products for assessing frictional forces. Part of the reason for this relates to physics—a sensor that is placed between a shoe and a subject's sock measures shear that may not accurately reflect the actual shear that skin experiences. In this regard, the presence of a sock can result in measurements that are underestimated by between 86% and 92%.[46] In other words, skin may experience shearing of 100 kPa, but the sensor may only detect 10 kPa! Coefficients of friction between sensor and sock, or between sock and skin, together with sock stretchiness, all affect the accuracy of these measurements. The ability for future in-shoe shear sensor technologies to address the effect of sock material is still an open question.

Although sock materials may have some effect on pressure readings, the influence is likely minimal. For this reason, most commercial efforts to develop stress sensors have focused on pressure as opposed to shear. Novel GmbH, Munich, Germany, with U.S. offices in St. Paul, MN, is generally recognized as the technical and market leader in plantar pressure measurement systems. Comparisons between Novel's technology and other commercial systems (**Table 1**) highlight the reasons for their popularity in foot ulceration studies. They offer both platform (Emed) and in-shoe (Pedar) devices that come in a variety of models that are based on a well-established capacitive sensor system. This approach results in a system that shows excellent linearity and hysteresis characteristics. The Pedar system provides highly conforming elastic insole pads that cover the whole plantar surface or sensor pads for the dorsal, medial, or lateral areas of the foot. Insole pads are available in various shoe sizes that can provide up to 1024 sensors, which can be scanned at a rate of 20,000 sensors per second.

CHARCOT ARTHROPATHY AND FOOT ULCERATION

As evidenced by the above information, DFUs are one of the most common complications of diabetes mellitus. Another complication of diabetes that is important for physicians is the development of Charcot arthropathy. Although Charcot arthropathy of the foot is not as prevalent as DFU, approximately 35% of people with diabetes and peripheral neuropathy develop Charcot.[47] The disease outcomes for DFU and Charcot are as equally devastating to the patient.

Charcot arthropathy of the foot is a devastating degenerative disorder that derives from the dysregulation of the cardiovascular, musculoskeletal, and neurologic system. Charcot is characterized as a progressive degradation of the midfoot joint (**Fig. 6**). If left untreated, the disease can progress to ulceration (DFU), midfoot arch collapse, infection, amputation, or death. Current clinical evaluation for Charcot consists of temperature measurements on each foot, x-ray imaging, and clinical observations (swelling, redness, etc.).[24] Some have suggested using CT scans to track bone mineral density (BMD) and potentially identify those at risk for developing Charcot from peripheral neuropathy. These studies were able to diagnose those who already developed Charcot and predicted Charcot development at 14%.[48]

The exact etiology of Charcot development is not completely understood. Multiple theories exist; however, none have been concretely determined as the sole rationale for Charcot development.[49] The one clinical consensus that exists is the presence of inflammation before the radiological presentation and concrete development.

In addition to similar disease development between DFU and Charcot, (the dysregulation of multiple body systems and a previous peripheral neuropathy diagnosis), DFU and Charcot are also inherently related. For example, a person with diabetes and peripheral who have had a previous diagnosis of foot ulcers developed Charcot at a rate of 18%.[50]

Recent advances in Charcot and DFU research have pointed to a similar methodology for potential monitoring and diagnosis, the use of pressure and shear measurements underneath the midfoot. Multiple studies have illustrated the potentiality of the usefulness of using pressure and shear in clinical evaluation for both DFU and Charcot development.[28,29,51–53]

FUTURE RESEARCH IN FOOT ULCERATION MONITORING

The future of DFU research is focused on prevention, early detection, and accurate intervention. This is currently achieved through the use of wearable sensors, AI/

Table 1
Selection of companies with products used to monitor foot pressure and/or shear

Company/Technology	Sensor Principle	Options	Comments
Tekscan	Conductive ink	Both in-shoe (F-Scan®) and platform systems.	In-shoe sensor array can be trimmed to fit shoe. High resolution grid of sensors.
Paromed	Hydrocell sensors	Pressure platform and the Parotec® in-shoe system	Foot pressure measurements are used for automated insole fabrication.
Materialize Motion (formerly RSScan)	Resistive sensors	The Footscan® system includes entry-level and advanced options.	Foot pressure measurements are coupled with foot shape data and used for automated insole fabrication.
Sensor Products Inc.	Piezo resistive elements	Tactilus High Performance Footplate	Data sampling can range from 200 to 400 Hz. Used for orthotics and ulcer studies.
Pressure Profile Systems (PPS)	Capacitance approach	Pressure systems for different body regions	The TactileMat has large pressure mapping surface area (220 mm × 450 mm)
XSENSOR Technology Corp.	Capacitance approach	Both in-shoe and platform systems	High-speed, high-resolution plantar pressure and gait measurement data.
Innovative Scientific Solutions	Optical approach	Platform allows for both pressure and shear measurements	Calibration challenges for shear sensors are overcome by measuring the relative change in the position of a polymer film.

Healthy Foot

Charcot Foot

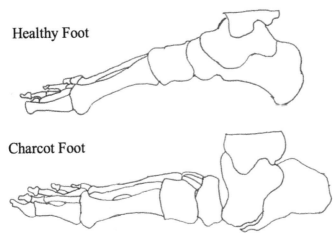

Fig. 6. Anatomic bone representation of a healthy foot structure compared with a Charcot foot structure.

machine learning, and smart technology. For example, some researchers are developing algorithms that can be applied to images of the feet. These algorithms can identify areas of the foot at risk for ulcer development; allowing the physician to focus clinical monitoring of that area.[54] In addition, the use of photographs and computer algorithms can allow for at home monitoring which could decrease the amount of lead time between DFU symptom onset and clinical intervention; thus, increasing patient outcomes.

Since there is a consensus among researchers that inflammation is a precursor to DFU, researchers are determining ways to measure temperature under the foot as an indicator of inflammation changes. Armstrong *and colleagues* has introduced a novel way to measure plantar temperature through a hand-held infrared temperature probe.[55] Others such as, Frykberg *and colleagues*, have approached plantar temperature monitoring through in-home smart mats (Podimetrics Mat) that can measure plantar temperatures and send the results through a cloud-based system to clinicians for review.[56] Doremalen *and colleagues* illustrated the viability of using smart-phone based infrared cameras to monitor plantar temperature for DFU detection.[57]

Wearable sensors are also on the horizon for DFU research. Siren Care are smart textiles made into socks that measure plantar temperature as a person walks and performs activities of daily living.[58] Wearable sensors can also be used to track pressure and shear stresses that are known to be a component in DFU development. Raviglione *and colleagues* suggested the use of smart socks (pressure sensor around a band) and a phone app to measure plantar pressure at home.[59] Due to the poor mismatch between areas of high plantar pressure and ulcer development, some researchers have suggested using shear as a metric to monitor for ulceration risk.[60] The ability to accurately measure shear forces under the foot using measuring techniques such as insole insoles is still in its infancy stages.

Finally, another facet of the future of DFU research is to increase patient compliance and wear time of interventions used to mitigate DFU development. Systems such as "@monitor" and Orthotimer are sensors integrated in prescription footwear that can measure the amount of wear time a patient has with their footwear while at home.[61,62] Some researchers have even used smart watches to provide alerts for adherence or instructions on better offloading to minimize plantar pressure peaks.

In-shoe sensors measure for adherence or pressure and connect to a smartphone app which then will send the data to the smart watch which then sends out the alert.[63,64]

SUMMARY

DFUs are a complex, multifaceted, and widespread complication of diabetes mellitus. Although there are a multitude of risk factors contributing to DFU development, pressure and (more recently) shear stresses are two biomechanical metrics that are gaining popularity for monitoring risk factors predisposing skin breakdown. Other areas of DFUs under research include plantar temperature measuring as well as monitoring wear-time compliance and machine learning/AI algorithms. Charcot arthropathy is another diabetes complication that has a relationship with DFU development, which should be monitored for development alongside DFU development. The ability to monitor and prevent DFU development and Charcot neuroarthropathy will lead to increased patient outcomes and patient quality of life.

CLINICS CARE POINTS

- Understanding the etiology of diabetic foot complications requires an interdisciplinary team approach.
- Diabetic foot ulceration is dependent on physiological, biomechanical and patient-specific factors.
- Skin breakdown is dependent on internal mechanical stresses as well as skin interactions with external surfaces. Both internal and external stresses are coupled with each other due to tissue properties and anatomical features.

DISCLOSURE

The authors have nothing to disclose.

ACKNOWLEDGMENTS

This work was supported by the T-32 NIH Training Grant: 5 -T32 - HL150389 – 03.

REFERENCES

1. Grennan D. Diabetic foot ulcers. JAMA 2019;321(1):114.
2. Armstrong DG, Boulton AJM, Bus SA. Diabetic foot ulcers and their recurrence. New Engl J Med 2017;376(24):2367–75.
3. Armstrong DG, Swerdlow MA, Armstrong AA, et al. Five year mortality and direct costs of care for people with diabetic foot complications are comparable to cancer. J Foot Ankle Res 2020;13(1):16.
4. Huang ZH, Li SQ, Kou Y, et al. Risk factors for the recurrence of diabetic foot ulcers among diabetic patients: a meta-analysis. Int Wound J 2019;16(6):1373–82 [published correction appears in Int Wound J. 2020 Apr;17(2):523].
5. Dubský M, Jirkovská A, Bem R, et al. Risk factors for recurrence of diabetic foot ulcers: prospective follow-up analysis in the Eurodiale subgroup. Int Wound J 2013;10(5):555–61.
6. Reiber GE, Smith DG, Wallace C, et al. Effect of therapeutic footwear on foot reulceration in patients with diabetes: a randomized controlled trial. JAMA 2002; 287(19):2552–8.

7. Monami M, Longo R, Desideri CM, et al. The diabetic person beyond a foot ulcer: healing, recurrence, and depressive symptoms. J Am Podiatr Med Assoc 2008; 98(2):130–6.
8. Waaijman R, de Haart M, Arts ML, et al. Risk factors for plantar foot ulcer recurrence in neuropathic diabetic patients. Diabetes Care 2014;37(6):1697–705.
9. Peters EJ, Armstrong DG, Lavery LA. Risk factors for recurrent diabetic foot ulcers: site matters. Diabetes Care 2007;30(8):2077–9.
10. Murray HJ, Young MJ, Hollis S, et al. The association between callus formation, high pressures and neuropathy in diabetic foot ulceration. Diabet Med 1996; 13(11):979–82.
11. Cavanagh PR, Simoneau GG, Ulbrecht JS. Ulceration, unsteadiness, and uncertainty: The biomechanical consequences of diabetes mellitus. J Biomech 1993; 26:23–40.
12. Ang L, Jaiswal M, Martin C, et al. Glucose control and diabetic neuropathy: lessons from recent large clinical trials. Curr Diab Rep 2014;14(9):528.
13. Boyko EJ, Monteiro-Soares M, Wheeler SGB. Peripheral Arterial Disease, Foot Ulcers, Lower Extremity Amputations, and Diabetes. In: Cowie CC, Casagrande SS, Menke A, et al, editors. Diabetes in America. 3rd ed. Bethesda (MD: National Institute of Diabetes and Digestive and Kidney Diseases (US); August 2018.
14. Noor S, Zubair M, Ahmad J. Diabetic foot ulcer—a review on pathophysiology, classification and microbial etiology. Diabetes Metab Syndr Clin Res Rev 2015; 9(3):192–9.
15. Mosa, Gehan & Elgohari, Amira & Elnassag, Bassam & Midan, Mahmoud & Attia, Mohammed & M Ahmed, Gehan. (2016). Center of Pressure Excursion and Stability in Diabetic Polyneuropathy. 117-123.
16. Toledo RC, Formiga CK, Ayres FM. Association between diabetes and vestibular dysfunction: An integrative review. Revista CEFAC 2020;22(1).
17. Kobayashi M, Zochodne DW. Diabetic neuropathy and the sensory neuron: New aspects of pathogenesis and their treatment implications. J Diabetes Invest 2018; 9(6):1239–54.
18. Henderson AD, Johnson AW, Ridge ST, et al. Diabetic gait is not just slow gait: gait compensations in diabetic neuropathy. J Diabetes Res 2019;2019:1–9.
19. Abri H, Aalaa M, Sanjari M, et al. Plantar pressure distribution in diverse stages of diabetic neuropathy. J Diabetes Metab Disord 2019;18(1):33–9.
20. Stess RM, Jensen SR, Mirmiran R. The role of dynamic plantar pressures in diabetic foot ulcers. Diabetes Care 1997;20(5):855–8.
21. Frykberg RG, Lavery LA, Pham H, et al. Role of neuropathy and high foot pressures in diabetic foot ulceration. Diabetes Care 1998;21(10):1714–9.
22. Schubert V, Héraud J. The effects of pressure and shear on skin microcirculation in elderly stroke patients lying in supine or semi-recumbent positions. Age Ageing 1994;23(5):405–10.
23. Everett E, Mathioudakis N. Update on management of diabetic foot ulcers. Ann N Y Acad Sci 2018;1411(1):153–65.
24. Bus SA. Innovations in plantar pressure and foot temperature measurements in diabetes. Diabetes/Metabolism Res Rev 2016;32:221–6.
25. Bus SA, Waaijman R, Arts M, et al. Effect of custom-made footwear on foot ulcer recurrence in diabetes: a multicenter randomized controlled trial. Diabetes Care 2013;36(12):4109–16.
26. Ulbrecht JS, Hurley T, Mauger DT, et al. Prevention of recurrent foot ulcers with plantar pressure-based in-shoe orthoses: the CareFUL prevention multicenter randomized controlled trial. Diabetes Care 2014;37(7):1982–9.

27. Yavuz M, Ocak H, Hetherington VJ, et al. Prediction of plantar shear stress distribution by artificial intelligence methods. J Biomech Eng 2009 Sep;131(9): 091007.
28. Caselli A, Pham H, Giurini JM, et al. The forefoot-to-rearfoot plantar pressure ratio is increased in severe diabetic neuropathy and can predict foot ulceration. Diabetes Care 2002;25(6):1066–71.
29. Davis B, Crow M, Berki V, et al. Shear and pressure under the first ray in neuropathic diabetic patients: Implications for support of the longitudinal arch. J Biomech 2017;52:176–8.
30. Davis BL. Foot ulceration: hypotheses concerning shear and vertical forces acting on adjacent regions of skin. Med Hypotheses 1993 Jan;40(1):44–7.
31. Yavuz M, Master H, Garrett A, et al. Peak plantar shear and pressure and foot ulcer locations: a call to revisit ulceration pathomechanics. Diabetes Care 2015 Nov;38(11):e184–5. Epub 2015 Sep 14. PMID: 26370381; PMCID: PMC4613917.
32. Bauman JH, Girling JP, Brand PW. Plantar pressures and trophic ulceration: An evaluation of footwear. J Bone Joint Surg 1963;45B:652–73.
33. Brand PW. Repetitive stress in the development of diabetic foot ulcers. In: Levin ME, O' Neal LW, editors. The diabetic foot. 4th ed. St. Louis, MO: Mosby; 1988. p. 83–90.
34. Delbridge L, Ctercteko G, Fowler C, et al. The aetiology of diabetic neuropathic ulceration of the foot. Br J Surg 1985;72:1–6.
35. Cavanagh PR, Ulbrecht JS. Biomechanics of the diabetic foot: A quantitative approach to the assessment of neuropathy, deformity and plantar pressure. In: Jahss MH, editor. Disor- ders of the foot and ankle. 2nd ed. Philadelphia: Saunders; 1991. p. 1864–907.
36. Masson EA, Boulton AJM. Pressure assessment methods in the foot. In: Frykberg RG, editor. The high risk foot in diabetes mellitus. New York: Churchill Livingstone; 1991. p. 139–49.
37. Thompson DE. Pathomechanics of soft tissue damage. In: Levin ME, O'Ncal LW, editors. The diabetic foot. 3rd ed. St. Louis, MO: Mosby; 1983. p. 148–1416 1.
38. Laing P, Deogan H, Cogley D, et al. The development of the low profile Liverpool shear transducer. Clin Phys Physiol Meas 1992;13:115–24.
39. Pollard JP, LeQuesne LP. Method of healing diabetic forefoot ulcers. Br Med J 1983;286:436–7.
40. Pollard JP, LeQuesne LP, Tappin JW. Forces under the foot. J Biomed Eng 1983; 5:37–40.
41. Tappin JW, Pollard J, Beckett EA. Method of measuring 'shearing' forces on the sole of the foot. Clin Phys Physiol Meas 1980;1:83–5.
42. Tappin JW, Robertson KP. Study of the relative timi ng of shear forces on the sole of the forefoot during walking. J Biomed Eng 1991;13:39–42.
43. Lord M, Hosein R, Williams RB. Method for in-shoe shear stress measurement. Jour- nal Biomed Eng 1992;14:181–6.
44. Huo M, Nicol K. 3-D force distribution measuring system. In: Hakkinen K, Keskinen KL, Komi PV, et al, editors. XVth congress of the international society of biomechanics: book of abstracts. Jyvaskylti, Finland; 1995. p. 410–1.
45. Cavanagh PR, Ulbrecht JS, Caputo GM. New developments in the biomechanics of the diabetic foot. Diabetes Metab Res Rev 2000;16(Suppl 1):S6–10. PMID: 11054880.
46. Tiell SM, Rezvanifar SC, Davis BL. The effect of frictional coefficients and sock material on plantar surface shear stress measurement. J Biomech 2021;127: 110682. Epub 2021 Aug 8. PMID: 34403854.

47. Rosskopf AB, Loupatatzis C, Pfirrmann CWA, et al. The Charcot foot: a pictorial review. Insights Imaging 2019;10(1):77.
48. Commean PK, Smith KE, Hildebolt CF, et al. A candidate imaging marker for early detection of charcot neuroarthropathy. J Clin Densitom 2018;21(4):485–92.
49. Botek G, Figas S, Narra S. Charcot neuroarthropathy advances: understanding pathogenesis and medical and surgical management. Clin Podiatr Med Surg 2019;36(4):663–84.
50. Fauzi AA, Chung TY, Latif LA. Risk factors of diabetic foot charcot arthropathy: a case-control study at a malaysian tertiary care centre. Singapore Med J 2016; 57(4):198–203.
51. López-Moral M, Molines-Barroso RJ, García-Morales E, et al. Predictive values of foot plantar pressure assessment in patients with midfoot deformity secondary to Charcot neuroarthropathy. Diabetes Res Clin Pract 2021;175:108795.
52. Lazzarini PA, Crews RT, van Netten JJ, et al. Measuring plantar tissue stress in people with diabetic peripheral neuropathy: a critical concept in diabetic foot management. J Diabetes Sci Technol 2019;13(5):869–80.
53. Perry JE, Hall JO, Davis BL. Simultaneous measurement of plantar pressure and shear forces in diabetic individuals. Gait Posture 2002;15(1):101–7.
54. Najafi B, Reeves ND, Armstrong DG. Leveraging smart technologies to improve the management of diabetic foot ulcers and extend ulcer-free days in remission. Diabetes Metab Res Rev 2020;36(Suppl 1):e3239.
55. Armstrong DG, Lavery LA, Liswood PJ, et al. Infrared dermal thermometry for the high-risk diabetic foot. Phys Ther 1997;77(2):169–77.
56. Frykberg RG, Gordon IL, Reyzelman AM, et al. Feasibility and efficacy of a smart mat technology to predict development of diabetic plantar ulcers. Diabetes Care 2017;40(7):973–80.
57. van Doremalen RFM, van Netten JJ, van Baal JG, et al. Validation of low-cost smartphone-based thermal camera for diabetic foot assessment. Diabetes Res Clin Pract 2019;149:132–9.
58. Reyzelman AM, Koelewyn K, Murphy M, et al. Continuous temperature-monitoring socks for home use in patients with diabetes: observational study. J Med Internet Res 2018;20(12):e12460.
59. Raviglione A, Reif R, Macagno M, et al. Real-time smart textile-based system to monitor pressure offloading of diabetic foot ulcers. J Diabetes Sci Technol 2017; 11(5):894–8.
60. Yavuz M. American society of biomechanics clinical biomechanics award 2012: plantar shear stress distributions in diabetic patients with and without neuropathy. Clin Biomech (Bristol, Avon) 2014;29(2):223–9.
61. Bus SA, Waaijman R, Nollet F. New monitoring technology to objectively assess adherence to prescribed footwear and assistive devices during ambulatory activity. Arch Phys Med Rehabil 2012;93(11):2075–9.
62. Lutjeboer T, van Netten JJ, Postema K, et al. Validity and feasibility of a temperature sensor for measuring use and non-use of orthopaedic footwear. J Rehabil Med 2018;50(10):920–6.
63. Najafi B, Ron E, Enriquez A, et al. Smarter sole survival: will neuropathic patients at high risk for ulceration use a smart insole-based foot protection system? J Diabetes Sci Technol 2017;11(4):702–13.
64. Abbott CA, Chatwin KE, Foden P, et al. Innovative intelligent insole system reduces diabetic foot ulcer recurrence at plantar sites: A prospective, randomised, proof-of-concept study. Lancet Digital Health 2019;1(6). https://doi.org/10.1016/s2589-7500(19)30128-1.

Biomechanical Implications of Congenital Conditions of the Foot/Ankle

Karen M. Kruger, PhD[a,b,*], Peter A. Smith, MD[a], Joseph J. Krzak, PT, PhD[a,c]

KEYWORDS

- Pediatric • Segmental foot model • Cerebral palsy • Charcot-Marie-Tooth
- Clubfoot

KEY POINTS

- Segmental foot and ankle modeling is commonly included during instrumented gait analysis to quantify foot and ankle motion during ambulation.
- It is important to understand technical differences in reported models and how this can alter clinical interpretation of results.
- Segmental foot and ankle models have been used to characterize atypical foot and ankle motion, identify clinically relevant subgroups among pediatric populations, quantify postoperative outcomes, and explain variability in healthy populations.
- Biplane fluoroscopy is a promising, emerging technology that provides a means to track the 3D motion of foot and ankle joints not amenable to traditional motion-capture strategies.

INTRODUCTION

Instrumented gait analysis (IGA) is a commonly used tool for treatment planning of complex congenital foot conditions.[1] IGA typically includes collection of temporal-spatial, kinematic, kinetic, and electromyographic data during locomotion combined with a physical examination. IGA has been extensively used across ages and pathologic conditions to guide clinicians' decisions about appropriate interventions, providing objective data about the efficacy of orthopedic surgery, and longitudinally tracking the progression of various disease processes.[2] Most commonly, kinematics

[a] Motion Analysis Center, Shriners Children's Chicago, 2211 North Oak Park Avenue, Chicago, IL 60707, USA; [b] Orthopedic and Rehabilitation Engineering Center, Marquette University & Medical College of Wisconsin, 1515 W. Wisconsin Avenue, Milwaukee, WI, 53233, USA; [c] Physical Therapy Program, Midwestern University, College of Health Sciences, 555 31st Street, Downers Grove, IL 60515, USA
* Corresponding author.
E-mail address: karen.kruger@marquette.edu

Foot Ankle Clin N Am 28 (2023) 27–43
https://doi.org/10.1016/j.fcl.2022.10.003
1083-7515/23/© 2022 Elsevier Inc. All rights reserved.

foot.theclinics.com

are collected during IGA using spherical, noncollinear, retro reflective markers placed over specific bony prominences to track the motion of a segment in 3-dimensional space. The most commonly tracked segments include the pelvis, thigh, shank, and the foot.[3]

In most conventional gait models, the foot is assumed to be a rigid-body. It is well accepted that referring to the "foot" biomechanically as a single segment is an over-simplification of a structure that contains 28 bones, intricate articulations, and hundreds of ligaments and muscles.[1,4] Utilization of a single-segment model to represent foot motion during gait can potentially neglect to identify deformity within the foot complex. Moreover, even when abnormalities are identified within the foot and ankle segments, it is not possible to isolate the problem to a particular joint. During the last several decades, segmental foot models have been used as part of clinical gait analysis to identify atypical segmental foot motion during movement, plan surgical procedures, identify kinematic subgroups within a population, and measure the effectiveness of intervention(s) on improving foot and ankle motion.

A recent review by Leardini and colleagues[5] identified nearly 40 segmental foot models that have been used for clinical applications and differed in the number of segments, bony landmarks, marker set, definition of anatomic frames, and convention for the calculation of joint rotations. Only a few of these models have undergone robust validation studies. Therefore, caution should be used when interpreting segmental foot results and comparing results across models.

It is also important to understand that axis alignment based on skin markers in a segmental foot model may not necessarily correspond to underlying skeletal anatomy and that misalignment is likely to be compounded in cases of foot deformity. Recent model-based analysis of the calcaneus has shown that the orientation of the hindfoot is highly variable, and markers placed posterior calcaneal tuberosity alone, as is the case with most segmental foot models, may not represent the orientation of the body of the calcaneus.[6] The Milwaukee Foot model (MFM) has been identified as one of the 4 most widely published segmental foot models[7] and has been validated for use in the pediatric population.[8,9]

An important processing step when modeling human biomechanics is neutral referencing. During neutral referencing, data collection from the static trial is used to mathematically link the orientation of the surface markers to the underlying skeletal anatomy. Neutral referencing using traditional methods assumes that the markers placed on the skin accurately represent the position, orientation, and motion of the underlying skeletal anatomy. This can be difficult in the hindfoot because reliable bony landmarks do not exist on the calcaneus to adequately represent orientation of this segment. The MFM addresses this problem by using a series of weight-bearing, roentographic offset measurements in anterior/posterior, lateral, and a unique hindfoot coronal view for the purpose of neutral referencing.[10] These measurements are used to reorient the embedded segmental local coordinate axes so that they align with the underlying skeletal segments. These radiographic measures are extremely important to the calculation of not only the offsets of the individual segments but also affect the kinematics of other segments and planes of motion.[11] The importance of using this type of technique becomes more apparent when dealing with significant foot deformities found in the pediatric populations where neutral alignment may be impossible to obtain talipes equinovarus (clubfoot), Charcot-Marie-Tooth, and plano-valgus/equinovarus associated with cerebral palsy. To calculate intersegmental angles, the segmental kinematics are expressed with the tibia referenced to the global coordinate axes. The remaining segments are represented in a distal relative to the next proximal segment relationship.

KINEMATIC FOOT TYPES

Early study in segmental foot models showed large standard deviations or "gray bands" in hindfoot and forefoot motion.[9] This has been shown to be a result of different foot types within the population. Root and colleagues described the following foot types in the healthy adult population based on specific morphologic features: rectus (well-aligned hindfoot and forefoot), planus (low arch, valgus hindfoot, and/or varus forefoot), and cavus (high arch, varus hindfoot, and/or valgus forefoot).[12] Further investigation of these foot types has identified that these foot types not only had unique static morphologic features but also unique biomechanical characteristics during ambulation.[13–15]

Our group previously investigated segmental kinematic differences between these foot types and results showed triplanar differences in hindfoot and forefoot motion (**Fig. 1**).[16] The cavus group showed increased dorsiflexion and inversion in the hindfoot and increased plantarflexion, valgus, and adduction in the forefoot when compared with the rectus group. The planus group was shown to have less dorsiflexion, more eversion, and more external rotation in the hindfoot and less plantarflexion and increased varus in the forefoot. Additionally, individuals with a planus foot type had a premature peak velocity toward coronal varus and early transition toward valgus, likely due to a deficient windless mechanism. Planus feet have also been associated with increased first ray mobility (**Fig. 2**).[17] Understanding the biomechanics of these foot types within the healthy asymptomatic population is critical to the proper care of patients with a variety of foot deformities or orthopedic impairments. Identification of these unique kinematics among foot types explains the variability among healthy adults and could result in the development of multiple reference ranges for identification of atypical motion and goal setting during clinical care, as well as identifying an appropriate comparison group for future clinical research studies.

CASE EXAMPLES

Our hospital uses this model as part of standard of care clinical IGA for children with congenital foot conditions. Case examples of 4 conditions are presented below.

CASE 1: MYELOMENINGOCELE—EQUINOCAVOVARUS FOOT

A 12-year-old girl presented with an equinocavovarus foot deformity, which was refractory to conservative management (**Fig. 3**). She walked independently without any braces and exhibited significant drop foot, varus foot position, and persistent

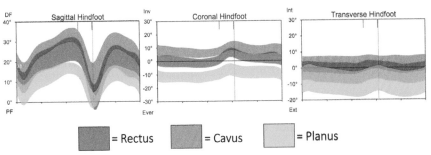

Fig. 1. Hindfoot kinematics of rectus, cavus, and planus foot types.

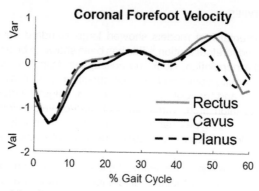

Fig. 2. Mean coronal forefoot angular velocities (with respect to the hindfoot) among the rectus, planus, and cavus groups across the stance phase of the gait cycle (0%–60%). (Karen M. Kruger, Adam Graf, Ann Flanagan, Benjamin D. McHenry, Haluk Altiok, Peter A. Smith, Gerald F. Harris, Joseph J. Krzak, Segmental foot and ankle kinematic differences between rectus, planus, and cavus foot types, Journal of Biomechanics, 94, 2019, 180–186, https://doi.org/10.1016/j.jbiomech.2019.07.032.)

knee flexion on the left foot. Although there was no foot pain, she experienced occasional tripping and falling. Her surgical history included tethered cord release at 5 months of age, and a repeat tethered cord release when she was 11.5 years old. Following the second detethering procedure, the patient began experiencing occasional shin pain.

Physical examination included the following findings:

- Rigid hindfoot varus (both weight-bearing and nonweight-bearing)
- Rigid midfoot cavus (both weight-bearing and nonweight-bearing) that increased with dorsiflexion of the hallux
- Active, antigravity, ankle dorsiflexion with forefoot deviation into varus

Segmental foot and ankle kinematics (**Fig. 4**) showed:

- Sagittal plane: Increased mean hindfoot dorsiflexion during stance phase, increased forefoot plantarflexion throughout swing phase (ie, drop foot), increased forefoot excursion throughout the gait cycle.
- Coronal plane: Increased mean hindfoot inversion, increased mean forefoot varus, and increased coronal forefoot excursion throughout the gait cycle.
- Transverse plane: Increased mean hindfoot internal rotation and increased forefoot adduction throughout the gait cycle.

Based on these findings, the surgical plan included a calcaneal osteotomy, midfoot dorsal closing wedge osteotomy, plantar fascia release, Achilles tendon lengthening, and split anterior tibialis tendon transfer.

Postoperative findings (1 year following surgery) included the following improvements:

- Sagittal plane: Reduction in hindfoot dorsiflexion, forefoot plantar flexion (ie, reduced cavus and drop foot), and overall forefoot excursion.
- Coronal plane: Forefoot excursion and alignment approximating healthy controls.
- Transverse plane: Improved forefoot adduction throughout the gait cycle.

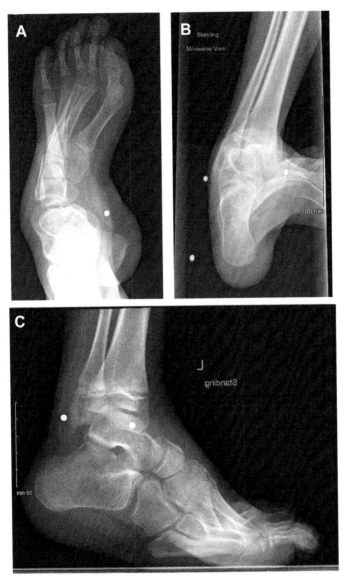

Fig. 3. Radiographs for case example #1. (*A*) A/P view, (*B*) Milwaukee view, and (*C*) Lateral view.

CASE 2: CHARCOT-MARIE-TOOTH (CMT) - CAVOVARUS FOOT

A 14-year-old girl diagnosed with Charcot-Marie-Tooth presented with bilateral cavovarus foot and fatigue and foot pain with walking (**Fig. 5**). Her complaints began around age 6 when the foot deformity was first noticed, and at the time of the preoperative evaluation, reported that she was able to walk for 5 to 10 minutes before feeling pain and fatigue.

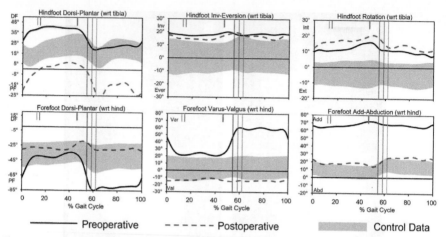

Fig. 4. Segmental foot kinematics preoperatively and 1 year postoperatively. Hindfoot measure is hindfoot segment motion relative to tibia and forefoot measure is forefoot relative to hindfoot.

Physical examination findings revealed:

- Rigid hindfoot varus (both weight-bearing and nonweight-bearing)
- Midfoot cavus (both weight-bearing and nonweight-bearing) that increased with dorsiflexion of the hallux
- Weakness of ankle dorsiflexors, evertors, and plantarflexors.

Segmental foot and ankle kinematics (**Fig. 6**) showed:

- Sagittal plane: Increased progression toward and persistence of hindfoot/forefoot plantar flexion from third rocker throughout swing phase.
- Coronal plane: Increased peak hindfoot inversion and increased progression/excursion into varus at the forefoot from third rocker throughout swing phase.
- Transverse plane: Increased mean hindfoot external rotation and forefoot adduction. Forefoot adduction continues to progress throughout swing phase. Together, this data supports progressive supination from third rocker throughout swing phase.

Based on these findings, the surgical plan included a posterior tibialis transfer dorsally, plantar fascia release, and a calcaneal sliding osteotomy.

Postoperative segmental foot and ankle kinematic plots 1 year following surgery revealed significant improvement in her cavovarus posture during the gait cycle, particularly in improved hindfoot varus, rotation, and forefoot adduction.

CASE 3: CLUBFOOT

The patient was an 8-year-old boy with a diagnosis of bilateral idiopathic congenital talipes equinovarus (clubfoot) deformities and generalized hypotonia and weakness (**Fig. 7**). He initially underwent Ponseti casting, bilateral heel cord tenotomies, and used Denis-Browne type shoes and bar. He later underwent surgical correction for residual deformity that included tibial derotational osteotomies and calcaneal osteotomies. At the time of the most recent evaluation, he reported persistent bilateral foot pain and an overcorrected clubfoot.

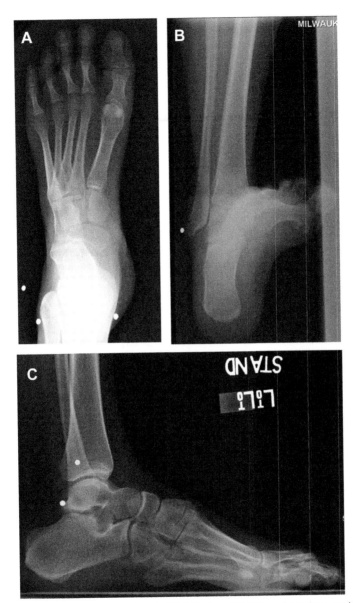

Fig. 5. Radiographs for case example #2. (*A*) A/P view, (*B*) Milwaukee view, and (*C*) lateral view.

Physical examination findings revealed:

- Mild plantar flexor tightness (gastrocnemius and soleus)
- Rigid hindfoot valgus (both weight-bearing and nonweight-bearing)
- Flexible forefoot abductus

Segmental foot kinematics showed (**Fig. 8**):

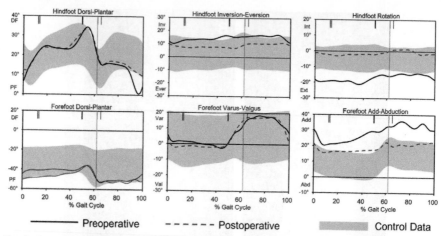

Fig. 6. Segmental foot kinematics preoperatively and 1 year postoperatively. Hindfoot measure is hindfoot segment motion relative to tibia and forefoot measure is forefoot relative to hindfoot.

- Sagittal plane: Decreased calcaneal pitch on A/P radiograph. Decreased mean hindfoot dorsiflexion throughout the gait cycle and decreased hindfoot/forefoot excursion during third rocker indicate lack of any type of push-off.
- Coronal plane: Persistent hindfoot eversion and forefoot varus (relative to the hindfoot)
- Transverse plane: Persistent external foot progression angle resulting from combined hindfoot external rotation and forefoot abduction.

Based on these findings, the surgical plan included a calcaneal sliding osteotomy was performed to improve his foot position.

CASE 4: CEREBRAL PALSY—PLANOVALGUS FOOT

The patient was a 16-year-old girl diagnosed with spastic diplegic cerebral palsy. At the time of the preoperative evaluation, she ambulated using bilateral forearm crutches and reported increased tripping and falling (**Fig. 9**). She has a history of previous lower extremity surgeries including a right foot STA-peg procedure with gastrocnemius lengthening, a right tibial and fibular derotational osteotomies and plating with short leg casting.
Physical examination findings revealed:

- Plantar flexor tightness, particularly of the gastrocnemius, with confirmed midfoot break
- Flexible forefoot abductus

Segmental foot kinematics showed (**Fig. 10**):

- Sagittal plane: Persistent hindfoot plantar flexion, decreased forefoot plantar flexion, and decreased overall segmental excursions indicate a midfoot break.
- Transverse plane: Persistent increased forefoot abduction throughout the gait cycle.

To improve the foot position, a gastrocnemius lengthening and lateral column lengthening (LCL) were performed. Postoperative segmental foot kinematics showed significant improvements to her forefoot abduction.

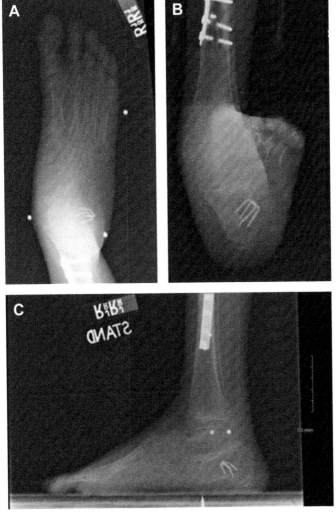

Fig. 7. Radiographs for case example #4. (*A*) A/P view, (*B*) Milwaukee view, and (*C*) lateral view.

POPULATION-BASED ANALYSES

Segmental foot models have been successfully applied to several populations of congenital foot conditions.[5] These models have been used to identify atypical segmental foot motion of specific pathologic conditions, identify kinematic subgroups within a population, and measure the effectiveness of intervention(s) on improving foot and ankle motion.

Clubfoot

The Ponseti method is the most common treatment option for clubfoot, which consists of serial foot manipulation and placement of stretching casts, followed by Achilles tenotomy and finally foot abduction bracing to maintain the correction.[18] Before the

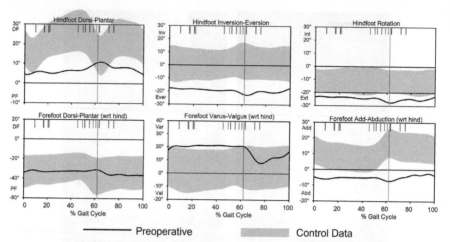

Fig. 8. Segmental foot kinematics preoperatively. Hindfoot measure is hindfoot segment motion relative to tibia and forefoot measure is forefoot relative to hindfoot.

Ponseti method, the comprehensive clubfoot surgical release was the standard of care and still is used for individuals when nonoperative management fails. The Ponseti method has shown favorable results including plantigrade feet with good overall function including sports participation but there remains a high rate of relapse and may require more invasive surgery for correction.[19,20] Segmental foot models have been used to classify children following these treatments. Residual internal foot progression (intoeing gait) is a commonly recognized clinical problem. Theologis and colleagues used the Oxford Foot model to analyze a group of children who had previously had surgical correction of clubfoot. Results showed internal rotation of both the hindfoot relative to the tibia and forefoot relative to the hindfoot, indicating the intoeing resulted from deviations at both of these segments.[21] Results also showed increased range of motion of the forefoot in relation to the hindfoot as a compensation for decreased range of motion of the hindfoot in relation to the tibia. Children who had Ponseti treatment were also analyzed using the Oxford Foot model and showed decreased forefoot-to-hindfoot range of motion but normal hindfoot-to-tibia range of motion.[22] Results also showed that forefoot adduction was primarily contributing to residual/recurrent intoeing gait following Ponseti treatment.

Planovalgus

Pes planovalgus is characterized by an equinus deformity of the hindfoot, protonation of the midfoot and forefoot, and shortening of the lateral column.[23] In typically developing children, the disorder is often flexible and the arch is reconstituted with dorsiflexion of the hallux or with voluntary plantarflexion. Flexible flatfoot is often asymptomatic or causes minor discomfort to the foot and lower extremity, and is treated conservatively with supportive footwear or orthotics.[24] However, the condition can be rigid, evidenced by a persistent flat arch even during nonweight-bearing. These cases benefit from bracing or surgical intervention, which may consist of arthrodesis, calcaneal osteotomies with soft-tissue procedures, and subtalar arthroereisis.[25] Segmental foot models have been used to characterize this deformity in populations of children with and without neuromuscular involvement.

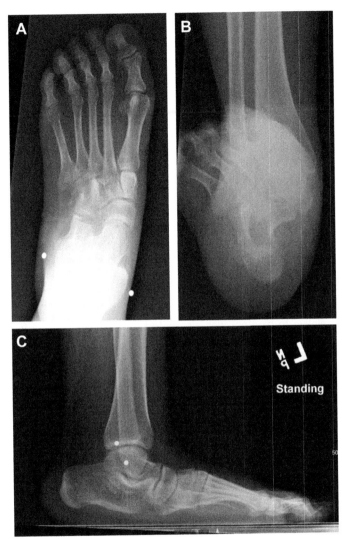

Fig. 9. Radiographs for case example #4. (*A*) A/P view, (*B*) Milwaukee view, and (*C*) lateral view.

Analysis of planovalgus feet without neuromuscular involved showed deviations including excessive hindfoot relative to forefoot eversion (valgus) and plantarflexion, reduced hindfoot flexion range of motion, and increased forefoot relative to hindfoot dorsiflexion and protonation. Contrary to clinical expectations however, there were no significant differences observed in forefoot flexion or hindfoot eversion ranges of motion.[26,27] Characterization of the midfoot in children with asymptomatic planovalgus showed the midtarsal joint was more dorsiflexed, everted and abducted than that in the control group, and showed reduced sagittal-plane range of motion.[28]

Segmental foot kinematics of children with planovalgus secondary to cerebral palsy have shown a combination of hindfoot plantarflexion and forefoot dorsiflexion, indicating a midfoot break occurring during walking.[29,30] Increased range of motion of

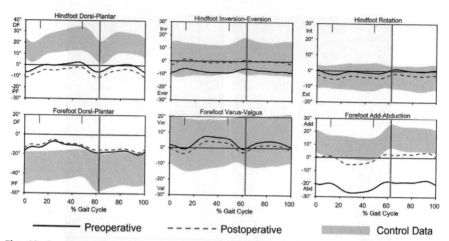

Fig. 10. Segmental foot kinematics preoperatively and 1 year postoperatively. Hindfoot measure is hindfoot segment motion relative to tibia and forefoot measure is forefoot relative to hindfoot.

the forefoot relative to hindfoot was also noted. Comparison of data from a single segment foot model and the Shriners Hospital for Children Greenville Foot Model showed the single segment model underestimated equinus across the ankle in the presence of a midfoot break and did not detect range of motion differences.[29]

Analysis of the hindfoot using skin-based motion capture can be challenging due to the lack of palpable landmarks on the calcaneus and as noted earlier, the axis by the segmental foot model may not necessarily correspond to underlying skeletal anatomy.[6] Analysis of this population using the MFM was able to show that within the planovalgus population, there is significant variability in coronal hindfoot alignment and there cares of hindfoot relative to tibia alignment in inversion, eversion, and neutral (**Fig. 11**).[30]

Kinematic Subgroups

Significant variability of segmental foot kinematics has been noted within specific foot pathologic conditions including equinovarus and planovalgus.[30,31] Identification of kinematic subgroups within these populations has been used to classify patients into subgroups based on specified gait parameters. Our group used principal component analysis (PCA) and cluster analysis to identify subgroups within children with cerebral palsy diagnosed with equinovarus and planovalgus.[32,33] PCA has been used to identify the most salient variables from large datasets while minimizing loss of valuable information. Once a dataset is reduced, cluster analysis can then be performed using K-means clustering on the principal components to identify subgroups of similar individuals. Analysis of children with equinovarus using these methods showed the presence of 5 kinematic subgroups within this population.[33] These subgroups presented with variable involvement ranging from primary hindfoot or forefoot deviations to deformity that included both segments in multiple planes. Analysis of a population of children with planovalgus revealed the presence of 4 kinematic subgroups.[32] These methods are intended to help standardize data interpretation and direct treatment since similar patients within a subgroup will likely benefit from the same intervention(s).

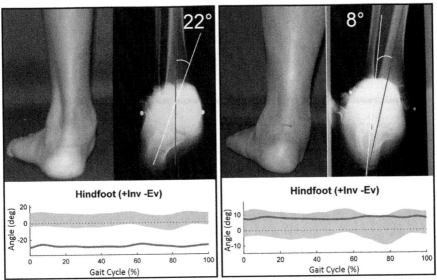

Fig. 11. Two sets of individual subject data illustrating the advantage of skeletal indexing in patients with planovalgus. One the radiographs, the calcaneus is defined as an ellipse, the tibia axis is defined by a dashed line, and the calcaneus axis is defined by a solid line. On the plots, black lines depict an average of the subjects' 3 trials; gray band indicates control average ± one standard deviation. (Karen M. Kruger, Katherine A. Konop, Joseph J. Krzak, Adam Graf, Haluk Altiok, Peter A. Smith, Gerald F. Harris, Segmental kinematic analysis of planovalgus feet during walking in children with cerebral palsy, Gait & Posture, 54, 2017, 277-283, https://doi.org/10.1016/j.gaitpost.2017.03.020.).

Long-Term Outcomes

There has also been interest in understanding the long-term biomechanical outcomes on surgeries performed for foot conditions in children. Although some treatments have been accepted standards of care for correction of foot deformities, the long-term prognosis for correction of foot deformity into adulthood has been well established in many cases.[34] Beyond atypical segmental alignment, position and motion, foot deformities are associated with gait deviations at more proximal segments, increased mechanical work and greater energy expenditure.[35] Therefore, there is a desire to identify postoperative impairments and limitations to guide future clinical decision-making for congenital foot conditions. These results can also provide clinicians and researchers the common residual and recurrent issues for these patients as they age.

Our group analyzed the long-term outcomes of LCL for treatment of planovalgus in children with cerebral palsy.[36] LCL is considered a robust, reliable operative procedure and is preferred over arthrodeses due to its ability to restore foot alignment while preserving joint motion.[37] Goals are to lengthen the calcaneus lateral column and push the navicular medially, reducing the talus over the calcaneus and straightening the midfoot/forefoot. We assessed 13 patients with cerebral palsy (average age = 24.4 ± 5.7 years) who had been treated with LCL an average of 15.3 years earlier using both a single segment foot model and the MFM. The ankle kinematics of the single segment model showed no differences during mid-to-late stance, despite the decreased calcaneal pitch observed in the radiographic assessment. However,

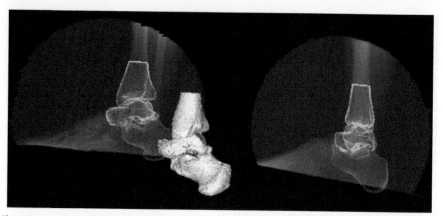

Fig. 12. View of fluoroscopy images and bone models of tibia, talus, and calcaneus.

the MFM results showed a combination of hindfoot plantarflexion combined with forefoot dorsiflexion throughout the gait cycle, indicating a midfoot break. There was also a flatting of several kinematic curves indicating reduced in range of motion. Additionally, the MFM kinematics showed residual forefoot abduction that was not appreciated with the single segment foot model.

Quantitative gait analysis with the MFM was also used to compare outcomes of adults who had received in either surgical treatment or Ponseti casting for treatment of clubfoot.[38] Patients in both the Ponseti and surgical groups had a plantar flexion shift in hindfoot kinematics and corresponding dorsiflexion shift in the forefoot kinematics throughout the gait cycle, with decreased hindfoot range of motion (ROM) from terminal stance to preswing. This shift was more significant in the surgical group. Both treatment groups also had a more external foot progression angle during preswing, a decrease in peak ankle power generation, and decreased dorsiflexion, inversion, and eversion strength with the surgical group showing larger deviations from the control group for all variables. These results reflect foot stiffness and altered biomechanics in adults who have been treated for clubfoot with either surgical release or Ponseti casting. The results of this study supported efforts to correct clubfoot with Ponseti casting and minimize surgery to the joints and highlights the need to improve methods that promote increasing joint range of motion and strength in these patients, which are important for adult function.

SUMMARY

Segmental foot models have been effective clinical tools as part of clinical gait analysis for congenital foot conditions and have been an important part of surgical planning by providing invaluable information on the dynamic function of the foot. They are subject to the limitation that in most published models, hindfoot motion is reported motion of the calcaneus relative to the tibia because the talus lacks reliable palpable landmarks to place external markers.[7] This therefore combines the kinematic contributions of the tibiotalar and subtalar joints, which are frequent sites of surgical concern with foot deformity.

Biplane fluoroscopy is an emerging technology that provides a means to track the 3D motion of these joints directly (**Fig. 12**).[39] It uses 2 radiograph images that are aligned with digitally reconstructed radiographs created from volumetric computed tomography (CT) scans, thus enabling visualization of specific bones during motion. This technique has been used to better understand tibiotalar and subtalar contributions of total ankle replacement,[40] flat feet,[41] and chronic ankle instability.[42] Use of biplane fluoroscopy in children has so far been limited because conventional CT is especially restricted in pediatric cases due to radiation dosage. Recent advances in cone-beam weight-bearing CT now allow for volumetric assessment of foot and ankle-bones with children with significantly less radiation exposure.[43,44] Current efforts are underway to develop standardized 3D anatomic reference frames for foot bones so that these new tools can be implemented across multiple sites.[45,46] These technologies hold large potential in increasing our biomechanical understanding of congenital foot and ankle disorders and how bone morphology relates to biomechanical function.

CLINICS CARE POINTS

- Segmental foot and ankle models are commonly used as part of IGA of complex pediatric foot conditions and can add invaluable information on the dynamic function of the foot and can contribute to clinical decision-making.

- Utilization of radiographic data with segmental foot and ankle models can increase model accuracy, especially in the presence of foot deformity.

- Unlike whole-body kinematics from IGA, segmental foot and ankle analysis was used to identify that there is more than one healthy control "gray band" of kinematics (ie, rectus, planus, and cavus foot types).

- There is noted segmental and planar variability (subtypes) within characteristic pediatric foot conditions that influence clinical decision-making.

DISCLOSURE

Authors have received funding from National Institute on Disability, Independent Living, and Rehabilitation Research (NIDILRR), United States and Shriners Children's, United States.

REFERENCES

1. Theologis T, Stebbins J. The use of gait analysis in the treatment of pediatric foot and ankle disorders. Foot Ankle Clin 2010;15(2):365–82. https://doi.org/10.1016/j.fcl.2010.02.002.
2. Wren TA, Gorton GE 3rd, Ounpuu S, et al. Efficacy of clinical gait analysis: A systematic review. Gait Posture 2011;34(2):149–53.
3. Davis R, Ounpuu S, Tyburski D, et al. A gait analysis data collection and reduction technique. Hum Mov Sci 1991;10:575–87.
4. Nester C. Lessions from dynamic cadaver and invasive bone pin studies: do we know how the foot really moves durig gait? J Foot Ankle Res 2009;2:18.
5. Leardini A, Caravaggi P, Theologis T, et al. Multi-segment foot models and their use in clinical populations. Gait & Posture 2019;69:50–9.
6. Zavatsky AB, Paik AMH, Leitch J, et al. Comparison of the hindfoot axes of a multi-segment foot model to the underlying bony anatomy. J Biomech 2019;93:34–41.
7. Leardini A, Stebbins J, Hillstrom H, et al. ISB recommendations for skin-marker-based multi-segment foot kinematics. J Biomech 2021;125:110581.

8. Kidder SMAF, Harris GF, Johnson JE. A system for the analysis of foot and ankle kinematics during gait. IEEE Trans Rehabil Eng 1996;4(1):25–32.

9. Myers KA, Wang M, Marks RM, et al. Validation of a multisegment foot and ankle kinematic model for pediatric gait. IEEE Trans Neural Syst Rehabil Eng 2004; 12(1):122–30.

10. Johnson JELR, Granberry WF, Harris GF, et al. Hindfoot coronal alignment: a modified radiographic method. Foot Ankle Int 1999;20(12):818–925.

11. Long JT, Wang M, Winters JM, et al. A multisegmental foot model with bone-based referencing: sensitivity to radiographic input parameters. Conf Proc IEEE Eng Med Biol Soc 2008;2008:879–82.

12. Root ML, Orien W, Weed JH. Normal and abnormal function of the foot. 1st edition. Clinical Biomechanics Corp; 1971.

13. Burns J, Crosbie J, Hunt A, et al. The effect of pes cavus on foot pain and plantar pressure. Clin Biomech (Bristol, Avon) 2005;20(9):877–82.

14. Hillstrom HJ, Song J, Kraszewski AP, et al. Foot type biomechanics part 1: structure and function of the asymptomatic foot. Gait Posture 2013;37(3):445–51.

15. Mootanah R, Song J, Lenhoff MW, et al. Foot Type Biomechanics Part 2: are structure and anthropometrics related to function? Gait Posture 2013;37(3):452–6.

16. Kruger KM, Graf A, Flanagan A, et al. Segmental foot and ankle kinematic differences between rectus, planus, and cavus foot types. J Biomech 2019;94:180–6.

17. Morgan OJ, Hillstrom R, Turner R, et al. Is the Planus Foot Type Associated With First Ray Hypermobility? Foot Ankle Orthop 2022;7(1). https://doi.org/10.1177/24730114221081545. 24730114221081545.

18. Dietz FR, Noonan K. Treatment of Clubfoot Using the Ponseti Method. JBJS Essent Surg Tech 2016;6(3):e28.

19. Cady R, Hennessey TA, Schwend RM. Diagnosis and Treatment of Idiopathic Congenital Clubfoot. Pediatrics 2022;149(2). https://doi.org/10.1542/peds.2021-055555.

20. Hosseinzadeh P, Kelly DM, Zionts LE. Management of the Relapsed Clubfoot Following Treatment Using the Ponseti Method. J Am Acad Orthop Surg 2017; 25(3):195–203.

21. TT N, HM E, T N, et al. Dynamic foot movement in children treated for congenital talipes equinovarus. J Bone Joint Surg Br 2003;85-B(4):572–7.

22. Mindler GT, Kranzl A, Lipkowski CAM, et al. Results of Gait Analysis Including the Oxford Foot Model in Children with Clubfoot Treated with the Ponseti Method. JBJS 2014;96(19).

23. Davids JR. The Foot and Ankle in Cerebral Palsy. Orthop Clin North Am 2010; 41(4):579–93.

24. Roye DP Jr, Raimondo RA. Surgical treatment of the child's and adolescent's flexible flatfoot. Clin Podiatr Med Surg 2000;17(3):515–30, vii.

25. Høiness PR, Kirkhus E. Grice arthrodesis in the treatment of valgus feet in children with myelomeningocele: a 12.8-year follow-up study. J children's orthopaedics 2009;3(4):283–90.

26. Saraswat P, MacWilliams BA, Davis RB, et al. A multi-segment foot model based on anatomically registered technical coordinate systems: Method repeatability and sensitivity in pediatric planovalgus feet. Gait & Posture 2013;37(1):121–5.

27. Saraswat P, MacWilliams BA, Davis RB, et al. Kinematics and kinetics of normal and planovalgus feet during walking. Gait & Posture 2014;39(1):339–45.

28. Caravaggi P, Sforza C, Leardini A, et al. Effect of plano-valgus foot posture on midfoot kinematics during barefoot walking in an adolescent population. J Foot Ankle Res 2018;11(1):55.

29. Maurer JD, Ward V, Mayson TA, et al. A kinematic description of dynamic midfoot break in children using a multi-segment foot model. Gait & Posture 2013;38(2): 287–92.
30. Kruger KM, Konop KA, Krzak JJ, et al. Segmental kinematic analysis of planovalgus feet during walking in children with cerebral palsy. Gait Posture 2017;54: 277–83.
31. Theologis T, Stebbins J. The Use of Gait Analysis in the Treatment of Pediatric Foot and Ankle Disorders. Foot Ankle Clin 2010;15(2):365–82.
32. Amene J, Krzak JJ, Kruger KM, et al. Kinematic foot types in youth with pes planovalgus secondary to cerebral palsy. Gait Posture 2019;68:430–6.
33. Krzak JJ, Corcos DM, Damiano DL, et al. Kinematic foot types in youth with equinovarus secondary to hemiplegia. *Gait Posture* 2015;41(2):402–8.
34. Miller F. Planovalgus Foot Deformity in Cerebral Palsy. Cereb Palsy 2018;1–40.
35. Stebbins J, Harrington M, Thompson N, et al. Gait compensations caused by foot deformity in cerebral palsy. Gait Posture 2010;32(2):226–30.
36. Kruger KM, Constantino CS, Graf A, et al. What are the long-term outcomes of lateral column lengthening for pes planovalgus in cerebral palsy? J Clin Orthopaedics Trauma 2022;24:101717.
37. Evans D. Calcaneo-valgus deformity. J bone Jt Surg Br volume 1975;57(3): 270–8.
38. Smith PA, Kuo KN, Graf AN, et al. Long-term results of comprehensive clubfoot release versus the Ponseti method: which is better? Clin Orthop Relat Res 2014;472(4):1281–90.
39. Cross JA, McHenry BD, Molthen R, et al. Biplane fluoroscopy for hindfoot motion analysis during gait: A model-based evaluation. Med Eng Phys 2017;43:118–23.
40. Lenz AL, Lisonbee RJ, Peterson AC, et al. Total Ankle Replacement Provides Symmetrical Postoperative Kinematics: A Biplane Fluoroscopy Imaging Study. Foot Ankle Int 2022;43(6):818–29.
41. Phan C-B, Lee KM, Kwon S-S, et al. Kinematic instability in the joints of flatfoot subjects during walking: A biplanar fluoroscopic study. J Biomech 2021;127: 110681.
42. Roach KE, Foreman KB, Barg A, et al. Application of high-speed dual fluoroscopy to study in vivo tibiotalar and subtalar kinematics in patients with chronic ankle instability and asymptomatic control subjects during dynamic activities. Foot Ankle Int 2017;38(11):1236–48.
43. B LJ, M I. Weightbearing CBCT, MDCT, and 2D imaging dosimetry of the foot and ankle. Int J Diagn Imaging 2014;1(2).
44. Holbrook HS, Bowers AF, Mahmoud K, et al. Weight-Bearing Computed Tomography of the Foot and Ankle in the Pediatric Population. J Pediatr Orthop 2022. https://doi.org/10.1097/bpo.0000000000002168.
45. Lenz AL, Strobel MA, Anderson AM, et al. Assignment of local coordinate systems and methods to calculate tibiotalar and subtalar kinematics: a systematic review. J Biomech 2021;120:110344.
46. Conconi M, Pompili A, Sancisi N, et al. New anatomical reference systems for the bones of the foot and ankle complex: definitions and exploitation on clinical conditions. J Foot Ankle Res 2021;14(1):66.

Role of Robotic Gait Simulators in Elucidating Foot and Ankle Pathomechanics

William R. Ledoux, PhD[a,b,c,*]

KEYWORDS

- Cadaveric gait simulation • Dynamic gait simulation • Stance phase
- Foot and ankle pathomechanics

KEY POINTS

- Testing of cadaveric feet has progressed from mechanical measurement of joint axes, to static testing of instances of the gait cycle, to dynamic testing of the entire stance phase of gait.
- Since the mid-1990s, dynamic cadaver gait simulators have been developed and used to address clinical questions by several groups around the world.
- Dynamic gait simulators have been used to study foot bone kinematics, joint function, muscle function, ligament function, orthopaedic foot and ankle pathologies, and total ankle replacements.

INTRODUCTION

Even with modern imaging techniques, such as biplane fluoroscopy and weight-bearing computed tomography, quantifying the mechanics of the foot and ankle presents a monumental challenge. With 28 bones, approximately 60 joints, and more than 100 ligaments, in addition to 20 intrinsic and 12 extrinsic muscles, there are numerous degrees of freedom to consider. Furthermore, the small intricate shape of the foot bones, along with closed-pack nature of the joints of the foot, makes quantifying foot bone motion very difficult.

EARLY CADAVERIC WORK

This challenge has partially been addressed by using cadaveric specimens to obtain measurements that are impossible to ethically generate on living subjects. Some of the

[a] Center for Limb Loss and MoBility (CLiMB), VA Puget Sound Health Care System, ms 151, 1660 South Columbian Way, Seattle, WA 98108, USA; [b] Department of Mechanical Engineering, University of Washington, Seattle, WA, USA; [c] Department of Orthopaedics & Sports Medicine, University of Washington, Seattle, WA, USA
* Corresponding author. Center for Limb Loss and MoBility (CLiMB), VA Puget Sound Health Care System, ms 151, 1660 South Columbian Way, Seattle, WA 98108.
E-mail address: wrledoux@uw.edu

Foot Ankle Clin N Am 28 (2023) 45–62
https://doi.org/10.1016/j.fcl.2022.11.005
1083-7515/23/Published by Elsevier Inc.

earliest studies include the work of John Manter, who used cadaveric feet to mechanically determine the axes of rotation of the subtalar and transverse tarsal joints.[1] He held part of the proximal foot fixed, while moving the distal portion with rods and pointers "bolted" to bones to trace joint motion. J.H. Hicks also used a mechanical technique to manipulate feet while determining the joint axes of rotation at the ankle, talocalcaneonavicular, and midtarsal joints, as well as for first and fifth ray motion.[2] The same author used cadaveric feet to explore the mechanics of the plantar aponeurosis and arch height, that is, the windlass mechanism.[3] These seminal studies laid the foundation for the work for Isman and Inman, who determined the axes of rotation of the ankle and subtalar joints for 46 cadaver legs with a more sophisticated, yet still mechanical, technique for foot manipulation.[4] Procter and Paul used the same optical/mechanical technique in the earlier studies[2,4] to determine the axis of rotation of the ankle and subtalar joints[5] and then developed 2 force equilibrium–based models of the hindfoot. These initial cadaver studies provided clinicians with a basic understanding of foot mechanics (e.g., extending the great toe will increase arch height) and axes of rotation (e.g., the subtalar joint is rotated $41 \pm 9°$ in sagittal plane and $29 \pm 8°$ in the transverse plane). However, these studies were not attempting to necessarily simulate any portion of the gait cycle, and this has limited the clinical utility of their findings.

STATIC CADAVERIC GAIT SIMULATION

After the initial cadaveric studies exploring foot function, the next level of complexity consisted of experiments designed to simulate pathology under static loading conditions. One common representative condition is the flat foot deformity; there have been several research teams who developed static cadaveric simulators to study this condition. Kitaoka and colleagues mounted 11 fresh frozen cadaver feet under 111 N axial load with no muscle forces and tracked the motion of the talus, calcaneus, and first metatarsal relative to the fixed tibia via an electromagnetic system.[6] Specimens were tested in midstance as normal and after a flatfoot model was generated by sectioning peritalar soft tissue structures. They were able to simulate a pathological foot with significant forefoot abduction, hindfoot eversion, and arch collapse. Using the same loading apparatus, this group next explored the effect of 2 reconstruction procedures (deltoid ligament reconstruction and flexor digitorum longus transfer) on cadaveric flatfeet during midstance.[7] The deltoid ligament procedure resulted in a return to normal arch height and recovered 10° of hindfoot eversion, whereas the changes due to the flexor digitorum longus transfer were minimal, and this procedure did not successfully restore the foot arch.

Niki and colleagues[8] expanded on this work simulating several instances in the gait cycle, including heel strike, midstance, and heel rise, with 8 cadaver feet. Specimens were tested as normal and again after a simulated flatfoot procedure had been applied, both with and without posterior tibial tendon loading. As with Kitaoko and colleagues, Niki and colleagues tracked static bone motion with electromagnetic sensors that were mechanically coupled to the bone of interest. They were able to generate small but statistically significant increases in hindfoot eversion with their flatfoot model. Their comparisons demonstrated that once soft tissues in the foot are attenuated, the tibialis posterior cannot overcome the soft tissue laxity.

Imhauser and colleagues conducted 2 studies looking at flatfeet and associated treatments. Using a custom loading device, they experimented on 6 cadaveric lower limbs; each was tested as a control and then as a flat foot at simulated heel off.[9] Axial loads were applied, but no muscles were loaded. The effects of 6 orthotic devices were explored, demonstrating that in-shoe orthoses stabilized the hindfoot and the medial longitudinal arch, but ankle braces were ineffective. The same group used a similar apparatus with the addition of a custom tendon loading device to develop and validate a flatfoot model.[10] Their work indicated that the tibialis posterior shifted the center of pressure anteriorly at heel off, whereas flat feet (with aberrant tibialis posterior forces) have a posterior center of pressure and abnormal loading of the medial structures of the foot.

A final static cadaveric flatfoot study to review is the work of Blackman and colleagues.[11] They developed a cadaveric flat foot model that involved the gradual attenuation of foot ligaments associated with posterior tibial tendon dysfunction.[12] The model demonstrated calcaneal eversion, talar plantarflexion and adduction, and navicular abduction during a simulation of midstance. Achilles tendon overpull was shown to increase the severity of the deformity.

This brief review on static cadaver simulations of the flat foot deformity has emphasized the findings to date while studying this clinical population. Researchers have developed flatfoot models from normal feet[6,8–11] and explored surgical treatments[7] as well as the effect of posterior tibial tendon loading,[8,10] orthotic devices,[9] and Achilles tendon overpull.[11] However, dynamic loading was not considered, as only static instances of the gait cycle were simulated, and therefore the utility of these studies is limited.

DYNAMIC CADAVERIC GAIT SIMULATION

The aforementioned static models, while enlightening, were fundamentally limited in their functionality and utility, as they only provided an insight for a single portion of the gait cycle. With researchers asking more detailed, nuanced questions and technology becoming more advanced, dynamic cadaveric gait simulators were a natural extension to the static apparatuses. Neil Sharkey's group, first at the University of California at Davis and then at Pennsylvania State University, pioneered these systems, but ultimately, sophisticated dynamic simulators were developed by numerous research teams around the world. For the most part, these simulators consist of customized electromechanical hardware specifically designed for controlling the interaction between a cadaveric foot and the "ground," but several of the more complex systems used off-the-shelf robots that were customized appropriately. Early systems often had constraints placed on some of the degrees of freedom (DoF), but more recent systems allowed for precise control of all 6 DoF. Most simulators also use actuator systems to apply appropriate muscle forces, and most have some kind of force or pressure plate for quantifying applied loads. Oftentimes, a retro-reflective kinematics system is used to track foot bone motion. Control strategies for manipulating the kinematics or kinetics of the system to ensure physiological loads on the cadaver are often very complex and proprietary. Furthermore, simulations are often limited (by the cadaver and hardware, respectively) to less than body weight forces and slower than gait speed velocities. In summary, inputs include the cadaveric specimen, the 6-DoF tibial kinematics, the ground reaction forces, and muscle forces. Outputs depend on the specific clinical question; they typically include foot bone kinematics and plantar pressure but may also be as specialized as joint stress or bone strain. Please note that although it is beyond the scope of this article to review the various simulators in any detail (e.g., types of hardware, control strategies, actuator mechanisms, types of tendon clamps, number of tendons actuated, DoF, simulation time, simulation load, and so forth), interested readers are invited to peruse Aubin and Ledoux's chapter on Cadaveric Gait Simulation for a more detailed, thorough review.[13]

Here is a list of the primary cadaveric gait simulators listed in order of the date of the first scientific article:

a. Pennsylvania State University, State College, Pennsylvania, USA[14-35]
b. Mayo Clinic, Rochester, Minnesota, USA[36-38]
c. Tubingen University Hospital, Tübingen, Germany[39-43]
d. University of Salford, Salford, United Kingdom and Iowa State University, Ames Iowa, USA[44-47]
e. Cleveland Clinic, Cleveland, Ohio, USA[48,49]
f. VA Puget Sound Health Care System, Seattle, WA, USA[50-61]
g. Katholieke Universiteit Leuven, Leuven, Belgium[62-66]
h. Hospital for Special Surgery, New York City, New York, USA[67-74]
i. Shanghai Jiao Tong University, Shanghai, China[75-77]

NONCLINICAL APPLICATIONS OF DYNAMIC CADAVERIC GAIT SIMULATION

Although cadaveric gait simulators have been used to investigate a wide range of clinical conditions, many initial studies emphasized the design, development, validation, and initial implementations of the simulators (**Fig. 1**).[17,36,37,39,49,51,53,62-67,75-79] Additional studies have used dynamic gait simulators to develop other hardware, including a fiber optic tendon force sensor,[24,80] bone strain measurement via strain gages or staples,[29] another fiber optic tendon force sensor,[81] a passive engineering mechanism for increasing tendon force,[57] and a shear wave speed–based tendon force transducer.[60] These studies are not discussed in any detail in this review, and interested readers are directed to Aubin and Ledoux for a more in depth discussion.[13]

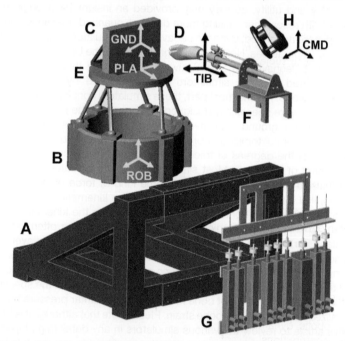

Fig. 1. Exploded view of the robotic gait simulator (RGS) developed at the VA Puget Sound with (A) surrounding frame; (B) motor attached to R2000 base; (C) mobile force plate; (D) cadaveric foot; (E) mobile top plate; (F) tibia mounting device; (G) tendon actuation system; and (H) 6-camera motion analysis system with only one camera shown. The coordinate systems shown are the ground (GND), plate (PLA), robot base (ROB), tibia (TIB), and motion analysis system (CMD). (*Reproduced from* Aubin et al.[53])

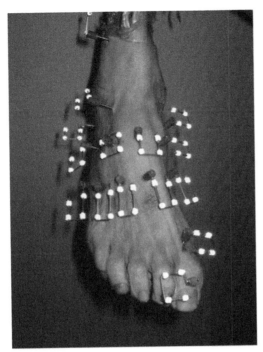

Fig. 2. Marker cluster technique used to track cadaver foot bone motion. The use of cadaveric tissue allows for invasive mechanical grounding of the markers to bones that would not be possible in living subjects. (C.J. Nester, A.M. Liu, E. Ward, D. Howard, J. Cocheba, T. Derrick, P. Patterson, In vitro study of foot kinematics using a dynamic walking cadaver model, Journal of Biomechanics, 40 (9), 2007, 1927-1937, https://doi.org/10.1016/j.jbiomech.2006.09.008.[47])

CLINICAL APPLICATIONS OF DYNAMIC CADAVERIC GAIT SIMULATION

Over the last roughly 3 decades, various groups have used cadaveric gait simulators to study various clinical aspects related to the foot and ankle. These areas have ranged from foot bone kinematics and joint function to muscle and ligament function. Studies have also covered a wide range of orthopaedic foot and ankle pathologies and treatments, in particular total ankle replacements. Hereafter, these various subtopics are highlighted with emphasis on a project or two that is of special interest clinically.

Foot Bone Kinematics and Joint Function

One early and fundamental use of cadaveric gait simulators was to track foot bone motion and joint function. Cadavers have afforded the use of rigid fixation techniques that would not be feasible with living subjects (**Fig. 2**). Sharkey and colleagues have used the robotic dynamic activity simulator (RDAS)[a] to (listed chronologically): (1) study the contributions of active (toe flexing musculature) and passive (plantar aponeurosis) toe flexion to forefoot loading (plantar pressure distribution)[21]; (2) report

---

[a] The various iterations of gait simulators developed by Sharkey and colleagues have also been referred to as the dynamic gait simulator or DGS. For the purposes of this review, the authors will not make any distinction between the RDAS or the DGS and instead use only the former term.

normal hindfoot (tibia, talus, and calcaneus) motion[27]; (3) quantify the accuracy of a generalized 3-segment skin-mounted kinematic foot model[32]; (4) determine the ability of skin-mounted foot models to diagnose pathologies such as cerebral palsy or stroke that cause aberrant muscle firing patterns[35]; and (5) explore the concept of midtarsal joint locking during heel strike and weight acceptance.[82] Nester and colleagues[47] demonstrated the errors associated with grouping foot bones together (rigid body assumptions) on foot kinematics. Some groups have generated normative foot bone kinematics for comparison,[51,77] whereas others have compared and contrasted normal with flatfoot kinematics.[38,72]

At the Cleveland Clinic Foundation, Lee and colleagues[48] studied the effect of diabetes on midfoot joint pressures. They tested 16 cadaveric specimens (8 control and 8 diabetic) on the Universal Musculoskeletal Simulator, which consisted of a rotopod, a force plate, a microscribe, a rotary actuator, 4 linear actuators, and custom LabVIEW code (**Fig. 3**). Tests were conducted at one-quarter the speed of gait and two-thirds the body weight. Four medial midfoot joint pressures (first metatarsocuneiform, medial naviculocuneiform, middle naviculocuneiform, and first intercuneiform) were measured dynamically during the simulated stance phase. On average, joint pressure was 46% higher in the diabetic feet and 3 of 4 joints (all but the first intercuneiform) had significantly higher joint pressures.

Muscle Function

Dynamic gait simulators have also been used to study the effect of muscle function on foot function. Ward and colleagues[48] explored how altered Achilles tendon forces can change the forefoot to hindfoot loading relationship.[83] Tibialis anterior tendon tears can be misdiagnosed because of extensor muscle compensation. To better

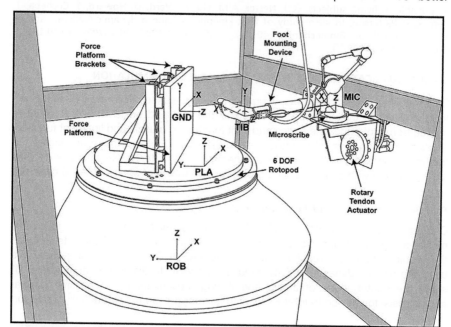

Fig. 3. Universal musculoskeletal simulator, consisting of a rotopod, a force plate, a microscribe, a rotary actuator, 4 linear actuators, and custom LabVIEW code. (*Reproduced from* Lee and Davis.[48])

understand this, one group has shown that tibialis anterior tendon dysfunction alters tarsal bone motion and plantar pressure in a predictable manner but that partial compensation can be achieved by other extensors (**Fig. 4**).[40] It has been supposed that multiarticular muscles function isometrically in order to transfer mechanical energy between joints. As such, the isometric function of the flexor hallucis longus was explored in 2 studies using the RDAS,[30,31] whereas a third study from this team examined isometric extrinsic toe flexor function during the stance phase of gait.[33] Using the tendon excursion method, a group from the Mayo Clinic calculated the moment arms of the 9 extrinsic muscles that cross the ankle joint.[84]

In a comprehensive article, Burg and colleagues[62] at the Katholieke Universiteit Leuven, Leuven, Belgium, demonstrated that the action of specific muscles alter foot joint kinematics. Their gait simulator consisted of a frame that supported pneumatic actuators that applied force to the tendons of the extrinsic foot muscles while the cadaver foot interacted with a force plate. They tracked motion of the talus, calcaneus, navicular, and cuboid, while varying muscle force to 4 functional groups of extrinsic muscles (**Fig. 5**). Data were collected in 3 static poses while individual muscle force was changed. (Yes, this is an example of a static simulation with a dynamic gait simulator.) They found that primary muscle group activity was the same for each bone and for the entire foot, for example, force applied to the triceps surae results in plantarflexion.

Ligament Function

Various groups have used cadaveric gait simulators to examine aspects of the relationships between ligaments and foot function. These studies have ranged from

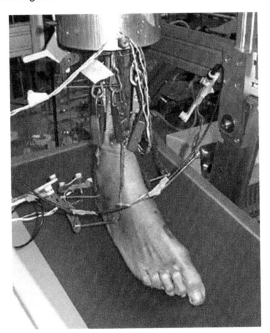

Fig. 4. Anterior-lateral view of a specimen mounted in kinematic and kinetic simulator during simulation of stance phase gait; this is shortly after heel strike during simulation of tibialis anterior muscle dysfunction, in which the specimen displays a drop foot position. Visible are the clamps and cable pulls, as well as ultrasonic motion analysis marker triangles. (*Reproduced from* Wulker et al.[40])

measuring spring ligament strain in intact feet and feet with posterior tibial tendon dysfunction during midstance,[85] to exploring the effect of partial release of the plantar fascia during stance phase,[86] to the peak pressure and pressure distribution in the ankle joint during stance phase.[43] The RDAS was used along with a fiber optic sensor to examine plantar aponeurosis force pattern and its relationship to Achilles tendon loads during normal gait (**Fig. 6**).[26] The RDAS was also used to explore how injuries to medial and lateral ankle ligaments can affect subtalar joint stability.[28]

Gait simulators have also been used to conduct ligament-based flatfoot studies.[38] In greater detail, the simulator developed by the Mayo Clinic consisted of a custom device that applied muscles forces to extrinsic tendons of the foot using 6 servo-pneumatic cylinders; vertical and fore-aft shear forces were applied, and tibial advancement was performed with additional servomotors, and the movements of foot bones were tracked with an electromagnetic system (**Fig. 7**). This device was able to apply specific time histories for vertical ground reaction forces and apply tendon forces based on the physiological cross-section areas and electromyography data from the literature. The flatfoot model was made by sectioning the peritalar soft tissue structures and by not applying any force to the tibialis posterior muscle. Motion of the calcaneus and first metatarsal was tracked relative to the tibia. This study found that the flatfoot cadaver feet had increased calcaneal and first metatarsal eversion and external rotation, demonstrating the effects of peritalar soft tissue disruption and lack of tibialis posterior force in a cadaver model that mimics the conditions found in living subjects.

Orthopaedic Foot and Ankle Pathologies

Since they were first successfully implemented in the mid 1990s, cadaveric gait simulators have been used to study and understand a broad range of orthopaedic foot

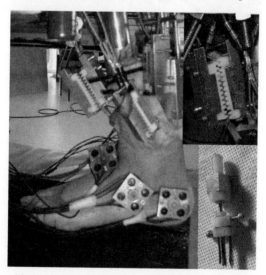

Fig. 5. Foot, mounted in the Katholieke Universiteit gait simulator. Custom built clamps are attached to the tendons of the 6 muscle groups. A detail of one clamp is shown in the top right of the image. The marker clusters, from which 3 are visible, are also present. A detail of an intracortical pin with a stabilizing device is shown in the bottom right corner. (*Reproduced from* Burg et al.[62])

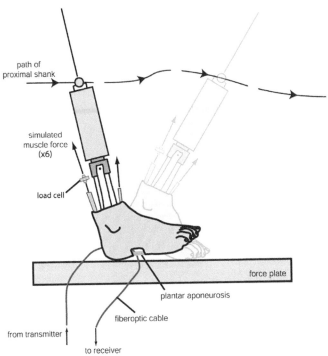

path of
proximal shank

simulated
muscle force
(x6)

load cell

force plate

plantar aponeurosis

fiberoptic cable

from transmitter

to receiver

Fig. 6. The dynamic gait simulator prescribed the path of the proximal part of the shank and the forces applied to the extrinsic tendons of 6 muscle groups: the triceps surae, tibialis posterior, flexor hallucis longus, flexor digitorum longus, peronei, and dorsiflexors (extensor hallucis longus, extensor digitorum longus, and tibialis anterior). In addition to fiberoptic light intensity, ground reaction forces were measured by a force plate and tendon forces were recorded with load cells attached in series. (*Reproduced from* Erdemir et al.[26])

and ankle pathologies and treatments. Neil Sharkey's team developed the RDAS and used it to quantify second and fifth metatarsal bone strain in normal and simulated fatigue conditions,[18] but they were unable to demonstrate that metatarsal microcracks were associated with bone strain.[20] The RDAS was also used to study the kinematic behavior of the ankle following malleolar fracture repair (**Fig. 8**).[23] Other studies have explored how ankle fusions alter foot joint kinetics and increase medial loading.[41] Other groups at the Mayo Clinic and Iowa State have used their respective gait simulators to explore the effects of foot orthoses on the work of friction of the posterior tibial tendon[87] and second metatarsal bone strain.[46] Prefabricated orthoses did not return posterior tibial tendon friction to normal levels, whereas both custom and prefabricated orthoses reduced bone strain. The VA Puget Sound research group developed a rotopod-based device, i.e., the robotic gait simulator (RGS), and correlated long second metatarsals with increased plantar pressure.[54] The RGS has also been used to quantify how second metatarsal shortening alters plantar pressure,[56] to determine the optimal angle of fusion for the great toe joint,[50] and to develop a flatfoot model.[52] The RGS was additionally used to explore the transfer of the flexor digitorum longus tendon to the navicular, medial cuneiform or the residuum of the tibialis posterior tendon (**Fig. 9**) in order to treat flatfoot deformity.[55] Studies mentioned earlier that used the RGS included the development of a passive engineering mechanism for increasing tendon force[57] and a shear wave speed–based tendon force transducer.[60]

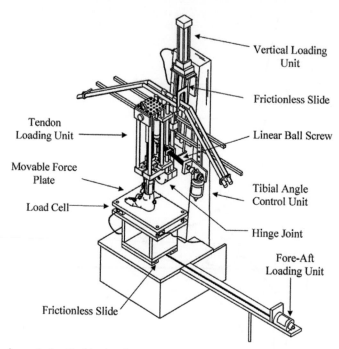

Fig. 7. The dynamic foot/ankle simulator. (*Reproduced from* Watanabe et al.[38])

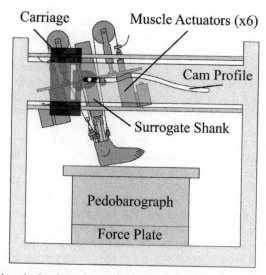

Fig. 8. The dynamic gait simulator (or robotic dynamic activity simulator) that was used to reproduce the stance phase of walking in cadaver feet. The foot is mounted to the actuator carriage, which progresses along a cam profile machined into a pair of guide plates. Stepper motor–driven linear actuators attached to the muscles by freeze clamps are mounted on the actuator carriage. The foot walks over a pedobarograph that sits directly on top of a force plate. (*Reproduced from* Michelson et al.[23])

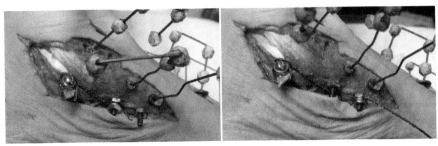

Fig. 9. Transected flexor digitorum longus tendon with custom fixation (via tendon clamp, string, and hanger bolt) to the (*left*) navicular and (*right*) medial cuneiform. (*Reproduced from* Vaudreuil et al.[55])

The Hospital for Special Surgery (HSS) has established a rotopod-based gait simulator with an important distinction from the VA Puget Sound's RGS. Namely, their robot is rotated on its side to align the cadaver foot properly with gravity. HSS used their system to determine that ankle arthrodesis increased adjacent foot joint kinematics[68] and to study the kinematics of the adjacent joints before and after sequential arthrodesis of the first, second, and third tarsometatarsal joints.[74]

In greater depth, the RGS was developed over a half-decade (roughly 2006–11) at the VA Puget Sound. It consisted of a force plate mounted to a 6-DoF rotopod. Cadaveric feet were mounted on the frame that supported the rotopod such that the force plate (i.e., the "ground") moved relative to a foot with a horizontal tibia. Nine extrinsic muscle tendons were attached to actuators that prescribed applied muscle force. Using custom-developed software, the motion of the force plate and the applied Achilles force were adjusted to obtain the required ground reaction forces. Plantar pressures and foot bone kinematics were quantified as the system outputs. As part of larger study into ankle arthrodesis and arthroplasty misalignment,[58,61] the RGS has been used to study the effect of anterior/posterior malaligned ankle arthrodeses on foot kinematics and plantar pressure (**Fig. 10**).[59] Changes in the center of pressure, peak plantar pressures, or joint ranges of motion were minimal; however, large anterior/posterior malalignments (6 or 9 mm) did shift the positions of multiple foot joints, for example, posterior malalignment of the ankle joint led to subtalar plantarflexion throughout stance phase. (As an aside, the team at the VA Puget Sound has nearly completed the development of the next-generation RGS. The main improvements include a rotopod upgrade, which allows for a vertical cadaveric tibia such that the feet can be correctly aligned with gravity. A new control architecture has been implemented, along with new tibial and force plate mounting systems, new muscle actuators, and a revised retro-reflective motion capture system.)

Total Ankle Replacements

After total ankle replacement, cadaveric gait simulators have demonstrated altered ground reaction forces[65] and modified bone kinematics.[66] The research team at the VA Puget Sound has quantified the effect of potential misalignment of the implant components on distal foot bone kinematics.[58,61] Another area of research related to total ankle replacements explored by the HSS team is the effect of a tibial joint position on distal bone kinematics.[69] This group also found that subtalar arthrodesis in cadaveric feet with total ankle replacements led to altered ankle and subtalar kinematics.[73] In combination with sophisticated computational models, the HSS team used

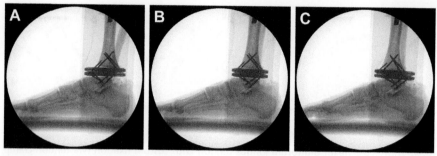

Fig. 10. Postoperative lateral radiograph of a specimen with the implanted custom fixture in the (*A*) 9A, (*B*) N, and (*C*) 9P alignments. A, anterior; N, neutral; P, posterior. (*Reproduced from* Imsdahl et al.[59])

dynamic cadaveric gait simulation to estimate the ankle joint loads in walking after ankle arthroplasty.[71]

In greater detail, the HSS cadaveric gait simulator prescribed tibial motions with respect to the ground while applying physiologic muscular loads to the 9 extrinsic tendons of the foot and ankle (**Fig. 11**).[67] The 6-DoF robotic platform moved a force plate relative to the tibia. Custom control software altered the force plate trajectory and the Achilles tendon force to match the target ground reaction forces. Subsequently, foot

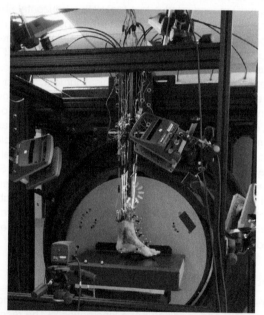

Fig. 11. The cadaveric gait simulator at HSS leveraged a 6-DoF robotic platform that moved a force plate about a fixed tibia, whereas 9 linear actuators applied prescribed loading profiles to the extrinsic tendons of the foot and ankle. Foot and ankle kinematics were quantified with an 8-camera motion capture system. (Reproduced from Saito GH, Sturnick DR, Ellis SJ, Deland JT, Demetracopoulos CA. Influence of Tibial Component Position on Altered Kinematics Following Total Ankle Arthroplasty During Simulated Gait. Foot Ankle Int. 2019;40(8):873-879.)

bone kinematics were recorded with a retro-reflective marker system. To date, this system is the most biofidelic, cadaveric gait simulator that has been developed.

Limitations of Dynamic Cadaveric Simulation

The primary limitation with all dynamic cadaveric simulators is that they inevitably fail to perfectly simulate gait. During normal walking, the ankle moves through a large range of motion, the ground reaction forces exceed body weight, muscle contractions lead to joint forces many times body weight, and numerous ligaments and muscles (both intrinsic and extrinsic) work in concert to stabilize the foot. All of this happens in about two-thirds of a second, making it extremely difficult to accurately replicate this behavior electromechanically with a cadaveric specimen. As such, simplifications are required; simulations are performed at slower velocities (~ 4 seconds or more for motion) at lower forces (one-quarter to one-half body weight), often with extrinsic muscles grouped together, and some simulators, but not all, limit the degrees of freedom that the foot can move. These concerns are mitigated by the fact that relevant trends are often seen even with the limited speeds and lower forces (e.g., a flat foot will still function as a flat foot even under less severe conditions).

DISCUSSION

Dynamic cadaveric gait simulators have been developed by numerous research teams around the world to address many clinical questions related to foot and ankle biomechanics. (A bulleted list of key findings is presented below.) Many simulators consist mainly of customized electromechanical hardware (Pennsylvania State University, Mayo Clinic, Tubingen University Hospital, Iowa State University, and Katholieke Universiteit Leuven), whereas others are based on off-the-shelf parallel robots, that is, either hexapods or rotopods (Cleveland Clinic, VA Puget Sound, Hospital for Special Surgery, and Shanghai Jiao Tong University). (Although not discussed in this review, several groups, including those at the Cleveland Clinic, VA Puget Sound, University of Virginia, and University of Utah, to name a few, are also exploring the use of serial robots to conduct cadaveric gait simulation. This technology is not widely published to date.) Although some simulators seem to have been retired, the systems in use at the VA Puget Sound and the Hospital for Special Surgery are still conducting clinically relevant research.

CLINICS CARE POINTS

- Diabetic subjects have higher joint pressures than control subjects.[48]
- Multijoint muscles function isometrically to facilitate the transfer of mechanical energy.[30,31]
- Peritalar soft tissue disruption is fundamental to the development of flatfeet.[38]
- Malalignment of ankle arthrodesis[59] or ankle arthroplasty[58,61] can alter distal foot bone kinematics.
- Subtalar joint arthrodesis in feet with total ankle replacements led to altered ankle and subtalar kinematics.[73]

DISCLOSURE

The author has nothing to disclose.

ACKNOWLEDGMENT

Department of Veterans Affairs grant RX002970

REFERENCES

1. Manter JT. Movements of the subtalar and transverse tarsal joints. Anatomical Rec 1941;80(4):397–410.
2. Hicks JH. The mechanics of the foot I. Joints 1953;78:345–57.
3. Hicks JH. The mechanics of the foot II. The plantar aponeurosis and the arch. J Anat 1954;88:25–31.
4. Isman RE, Inman VT. Anthropometric studies of the human foot and ankle. San Francisco: Biomechanics Laboratory, University of California, San Francisco and Berkeley; 1968. Technical Report 58.
5. Procter P, Paul JP. Ankle joint biomechanics. J Biomech 1982;15(9):627–34.
6. Kitaoka HB, Luo ZP, An KN. Three-dimensional analysis of flatfoot deformity: cadaver study. Foot Ankle Int 1998;19(7):447–51.
7. Kitaoka HB, Luo ZP, An KN. Reconstruction operations for acquired flatfoot: biomechanical evaluation. Foot Ankle Int 1998;19(4):203–7.
8. Niki H, Ching RP, Kiser P, et al. The effect of posterior tibial tendon dysfunction on hindfoot kinematics. Foot Ankle Int 2001;22(4):292–300.
9. Imhauser CW, Abidi NA, Frankel DZ, et al. Biomechanical evaluation of the efficacy of external stabilizers in the conservative treatment of acquired flatfoot deformity. Foot Ankle Int 2002;23(8):727–37.
10. Imhauser CW, Siegler S, Abidi NA, et al. The effect of posterior tibialis tendon dysfunction on the plantar pressure characteristics and the kinematics of the arch and the hindfoot. Clin Biomech (Bristol, Avon) 2004;19(2):161–9.
11. Blackman AJ, Blevins JJ, Sangeorzan BJ, et al. Cadaveric flatfoot model: Ligament attenuation and Achilles tendon overpull. J Orthop Res 2009;27(12): 1547–54.
12. Deland JT, de Asla RJ, Sung IH, et al. Posterior tibial tendon insufficiency: which ligaments are involved? Foot Ankle Int 2005;26(6):427–35.
13. Aubin PM, Ledoux WR. Cadaveric gait simulation. In: Ledoux WR, Telfer S, editors. Foot and ankle biomechanics. London: Elsevier, Limited; 2022. p. 351–63.
14. Ferris L, Sharkey NA, Smith TS, et al. Influence of extrinsic plantar flexors on forefoot loading during heel rise. Foot Ankle Int 1995;16(8):464–73.
15. Sharkey NA, Ferris L, Smith TS, et al. Strain and loading of the second metatarsal during heel-lift. J Bone Joint Surg - Am Volume 1995;77(7):1050–7.
16. Sharkey NA, Ferris L, Donahue SW. Biomechanical consequences of plantar fascial release or rupture during gait. Part I: Disruptions in longitudinal arch conformation. Foot Ankle Int 1998;19(12):812–20.
17. Sharkey NA, Hamel AJ. A dynamic cadaver model of the stance phase of gait: performance characteristics and kinetic validation. Clin Biomech (Bristol, Avon) 1998;13(6):420–33.
18. Donahue SW, Sharkey NA. Strains in the metatarsals during the stance phase of gait: Implications for stress fractures. J Bone Joint Surg Am 1999;81A(9): 1236–44.
19. Sharkey NA, Donahue SW, Ferris L. Biomechanical consequences of plantar fascial release or rupture during gait. Part II: Alterations in forefoot loading. Foot Ankle Int 1999;20(2):86–96.
20. Donahue SW, Sharkey NA, Modanlou KA, et al. Bone strain and microcracks at stress fracture sites in human metatarsals. Bone 2000;27(6):827–33.

21. Hamel AJ, Donahue SW, Sharkey NA. Contributions of active and passive toe flexion to forefoot loading. Clin Orthop Relat Res 2001;393:326–34.
22. Piazza SJ, Adamson RL, Sanders JO, et al. Changes in muscle moment arms following split tendon transfer of tibialis anterior and tibialis posterior. Gait Posture 2001;14(3):271–8.
23. Michelson JD, Hamel AJ, Buczek FL, et al. Kinematic behavior of the ankle following malleolar fracture repair in a high-fidelity cadaver model. J Bone Joint Surg Am 2002;84-A(11):2029–38.
24. Erdemir A, Hamel AJ, Piazza SJ, et al. Fiberoptic measurement of tendon forces is influenced by skin movement artifact. J Biomech 2003;36(3):449–55.
25. Piazza SJ, Adamson RL, Moran MF, et al. Effects of tensioning errors in split transfers of tibialis anterior and posterior tendons. J Bone Joint Surg Am 2003;85(5):858–65.
26. Erdemir A, Hamel AJ, Fauth AR, et al. Dynamic loading of the plantar aponeurosis in walking. J Bone Joint Surg Am 2004;86(3):546–52.
27. Hamel AJ, Sharkey NA, Buczek FL, et al. Relative motions of the tibia, talus, and calcaneus during the stance phase of gait: a cadaver study. Gait Posture 2004;20(2):147–53.
28. Michelson J, Hamel A, Buczek F, et al. The effect of ankle injury on subtalar motion. Foot Ankle Int 2004;25:639–46. SAGE Publications Inc.
29. Milgrom C, Finestone A, Hamel A, et al. A comparison of bone strain measurements at anatomically relevant sites using surface gauges versus strain gauged bone staples. J Biomech 2004;37(6):947–52.
30. Kirane YM, Michelson JD, Sharkey NA. Evidence of isometric function of the flexor hallucis longus muscle in normal gait. J Biomech 2008;41(9):1919–28.
31. Kirane YM, Michelson JD, Sharkey NA. Contribution of the flexor hallucis longus to loading of the first metatarsal and first metatarsophalangeal joint. Foot Ankle Int 2008;29(4):367–77.
32. Okita N, Meyers SA, Challis JH, et al. An objective evaluation of a segmented foot model. Gait Posture 2009;30(1):27–34.
33. Hofmann CL, Okita N, Sharkey NA. Experimental evidence supporting isometric functioning of the extrinsic toe flexors during gait. Clin Biomech (Bristol, Avon) 2013;28(6):686–91.
34. Okita N, Meyers SA, Challis JH, et al. Midtarsal joint locking: new perspectives on an old paradigm. J Orthopaedic Res 2013;46(15):2578–85.
35. Okita N, Meyers SA, Challis JH, et al. Segmental motion of forefoot and hindfoot as a diagnostic tool. J Biomech 2013;46(15):2578–85.
36. Kim KJ, Kitaoka HB, Luo ZP, et al. In vitro simulation of the stance phase of gait. J Musculoskelet Res 2001;5(2):113–21.
37. Kim KJ, Uchiyama E, Kitaoka HB, et al. An in vitro study of individual ankle muscle actions on the center of pressure. Gait Posture 2003;17(2):125–31.
38. Watanabe K, Kitaoka HB, Fujii T, et al. Posterior tibial tendon dysfunction and flatfoot: analysis with simulated walking. Gait Posture 2013;37(2):264–8.
39. Hurschler C, Emmerich J, Wulker N. In vitro simulation of stance phase gait part I: Model verification. Foot Ankle Int 2003;24(8):614–22.
40. Wulker N, Hurschler C, Emmerich J. In vitro simulation of stance phase gait part II: Simulated anterior tibial tendon dysfunction and potential compensation. Foot Ankle Int 2003;24(8):623–9.
41. Suckel A, Muller O, Herberts T, Wulker N. Changes in Chopart joint load following tibiotalar arthrodesis: In vitro analysis of 8 cadaver specimen in a dynamic model. BMC Musculoskeletal Disorders 2007;8:80.

42. Suckel A, Muller O, Langenstein P, et al. Chopart's joint load during gait In vitro study of 10 cadaver specimen in a dynamic model. Gait Posture 2008;27(2): 216–22.

43. Suckel A, Muller O, Wachter N, Kluba T. In vitro measurement of intraarticular pressure in the ankle joint. In. Knee Surgery. Sports Traumatology, Arthroscopy 2010;18(5):664–8.

44. Nester CJ, Liu AM, Ward E, et al. In vitro study of foot kinematics using a dynamic walking cadaver model. J Biomech 2007;40(9):1927–37.

45. Nester CJ. Lessons from dynamic cadaver and invasive bone pin studies: do we know how the foot really moves during gait? J Foot Ankle Res 2009;2:18.

46. Meardon SA, Edwards B, Ward E, et al. Effects of custom and semi-custom foot orthotics on second metatarsal bone strain during dynamic gait simulation. Foot Ankle Int 2009;30(10):998–1004.

47. Nester CJ, Liu AM, Ward E, et al. Error in the description of foot kinematics due to violation of rigid body assumptions. J Biomech 2010;43(4):666–72.

48. Lee DG, Davis BL. Assessment of the effects of diabetes on midfoot joint pressures using a robotic gait simulator. Foot Ankle Int 2009;30(8):767–72.

49. Noble LD Jr, Colbrunn RW, Lee DG, et al. Design and validation of a general purpose robotic testing system for musculoskeletal applications. J Biomech Eng 2010;132(2):025001.

50. Bayomy AF, Aubin PM, Sangeorzan BJ, et al. Arthrodesis of the first metatarsophalangeal joint: a robotic cadaver study of the dorsiflexion angle. J Bone Joint Surg Am 2010;92(8):1754–64.

51. Whittaker EC, Aubin PM, Ledoux WR. Foot bone kinematics as measured in a cadaveric robotic gait simulator. Gait Posture 2011;33(4):645–50.

52. Jackson LT, Aubin PM, Cowley MS, et al. A robotic cadaveric flatfoot analysis of stance phase. J Biomech Eng 2011;133(5):051005.

53. Aubin PM, Whittaker EC, Ledoux WR. A robotic cadaveric gait simulator with fuzzy logic vertical ground reaction force control. IEEE Trans Robotics 2012; 28(1):246–55.

54. Weber JR, Aubin PM, Ledoux WR, et al. Second metatarsal length is positively correlated with increased pressure and medial deviation of the second toe in a robotic cadaveric simulation of gait. Foot Ankle Int 2012;33(4):312–9.

55. Vaudreuil NJ, Ledoux WR, Roush GC, et al. Comparison of transfer sites for flexor digitorum longus in a cadaveric adult acquired flatfoot model. J Orthop Res 2014; 32(1):102–9.

56. Trask DJ, Ledoux WR, Whittaker EC, et al. Second metatarsal osteotomies for metatarsalgia: a robotic cadaveric study of the effect of osteotomy plane and metatarsal shortening on plantar pressure. J Orthop Res 2014;32(3):385–93.

57. Pihl CM, Stender CJ, Balasubramanian R, et al. Passive engineering mechanism enhancement of a flexor digitorum longus tendon transfer procedure. J Orthop Res 2018;36(11):3033–42.

58. Buckner BC, Stender CJ, Baron MD, et al. Does Coronal Plane Malalignment of the Tibial Insert in Total Ankle Arthroplasty Alter Distal Foot Bone Mechanics? A Cadaveric Gait Study. Clin Orthop Relat Res 2020;478(7):1683–95.

59. Imsdahl SI, Stender CJ, Cook BK, et al. Anteroposterior Translational Malalignment of Ankle Arthrodesis Alters Foot Biomechanics in Cadaveric Gait Simulation. J Orthop Res 2020;38(2):450–8.

60. Martin JA, Kindig MW, Stender CJ, et al. Calibration of the shear wave speed-stress relationship in in situ Achilles tendons using cadaveric simulations of gait and isometric contraction. J Biomech 2020;106:109799.

61. McKearney DA, Stender CJ, Cook BK, et al. Altered Range of Motion and Plantar Pressure in Anterior and Posterior Malaligned Total Ankle Arthroplasty: A Cadaveric Gait Study. J Bone Joint Surg Am 2019;101(18):e93.
62. Burg J, Peeters K, Natsakis T, et al. In vitro analysis of muscle activity illustrates mediolateral decoupling of hind and mid foot bone motion. Gait Posture 2013; 38(1):56–61.
63. Pootorc K, Natsakis T, Burg J, et al. An in vitro approach to the evaluation of foot-ankle kinematics: performance evaluation of a custom-built gait simulator. Proc Inst Mech Eng H 2013;227(9):955–67.
64. Natsakis T, Peeters K, Burg F, et al. Specimen-specific tibial kinematics model for in vitro gait simulations. Proc Inst Mech Eng H, J Eng Med 2013;227(4):454–63.
65. Natsakis T, Burg J, Dereymaeker G, et al. Inertial control as novel technique for in vitro gait simulations. J Biomech 2015;48(2):392–5.
66. Natsakis T, Burg J, Dereymaeker G, et al. Foot-ankle simulators: a tool to advance biomechanical understanding of a complex anatomical structure. Proc Inst Mech Eng H 2016;230(5):440–9.
67. Baxter JR, Sturnick DR, Demetracopoulos CA, et al. Cadaveric gait simulation reproduces foot and ankle kinematics from population-specific inputs. J Orthop Res 2016;34(9):1663–8.
68. Sturnick DR, Demetracopoulos CA, Ellis SJ, et al. Adjacent joint kinematics after ankle arthrodesis during cadaveric gait simulation. Foot Ankle Int 2017;38(11): 1249–59.
69. Saito GH, Sturnick DR, Ellis SJ, et al. Influence of tibial component position on altered kinematics following total ankle arthroplasty during simulated gait. Foot Ankle Int 2019;40(8):873–9.
70. Quevedo Gonzalez FJ, Steineman BD, Sturnick DR, et al. Biomechanical evaluation of total ankle arthroplasty. Part II: Influence of loading and fixation design on tibial bone-implant interaction. J Orthop Res 2021;39(1):103–11.
71. Steineman BD, Quevedo Gonzalez FJ, Sturnick DR, et al. Biomechanical evaluation of total ankle arthroplasty. Part I: Joint loads during simulated level walking. J Orthop Res 2021;39(1):94–102.
72. Henry JK, Hoffman JKim J, et al. The Foot and Ankle Kinematics of a Simulated Progressive Collapsing Foot Deformity During Stance Phase: A Cadaveric Study. Foot Ankle Int 2022;43(12):1577–86.
73. Henry JK, Sturnick D, Rosenbaum A, et al. Cadaveric Gait Simulation of the Effect of Subtalar Arthrodesis on Total Ankle Replacement Kinematics. Foot Ankle Int 2022. 10711007221088821.
74. Kim J, Hoffman J, Steineman B, et al. Kinematic analysis of sequential partial-midfoot arthrodesis in simulated gait cadaver model. Foot Ankle Int 2022. 10711007221125226.
75. Guo Q, Shi G, Wang D, et al. Iterative learning based output feedback control for electro-hydraulic loading system of a gait simulator. Mechatronics 2018;54: 110–20.
76. Wang D, Wang W, Guo Q, et al. Design and validation of a foot-ankle dynamic simulator with a 6-degree-of-freedom parallel mechanism. Proc Inst Mech Eng H 2020;234(10):1070–82.
77. Zhu G, Wang Z, Yuan C, et al. In vitro study of foot bone kinematics via a custom-made cadaveric gait simulator. J Orthop Surg Res 2020;15(1):346.
78. Nester C, Jones RK, Liu A, et al. Foot kinematics during walking measured using bone and surface mounted markers. J Biomech 2007;40(15):3412–23.

79. Aubin PM, Cowley MS, Ledoux WR. Gait simulation via a 6-DOF parallel robot with iterative learning control. IEEE Trans Biomed Eng 2008;55(3):1237–40.

80. Erdemir A, Piazza SJ, Sharkey NA. Influence of loading rate and cable migration on fiberoptic measurement of tendon force. J Biomech 2002;35(6):857–62.

81. Behrmann GP, Hidler J, Mirotznik MS. Fiber optic micro sensor for the measurement of tendon forces. Biomed Eng Online 2012;11:77.

82. Okita N, Meyers SA, Challis JH, et al. Midtarsal joint locking: new perspectives on an old paradigm. J Orthop Res 2014;32(1):110–5.

83. Ward ED, Phillips RD, Patterson PE, et al. 1998 William J. Stickel Gold Award. The effects of extrinsic muscle forces on the forefoot-to-rearfoot loading relationship in vitro. Tibia and Achilles tendon. J Am Podiatr Med Assoc 1998;88(10):471–82.

84. McCullough MB, Ringleb SI, Arai K, et al. Moment Arms of the Ankle Throughout the Range of Motion in Three Planes. Foot Ankle Int 2011;32(3):300–6.

85. Hansen ML, Otis JC, Kenneally SM, et al. A closed-loop cadaveric foot and ankle loading model. J Biomech 2001;34(4):551–5.

86. Ward ED, Smith KM, Cocheba JR, et al. 2003 William J. Stickel Gold Award. In vivo forces in the plantar fascia during the stance phase of gait: sequential release of the plantar fascia. J Am Podiatr Med Assoc 2003;93(6):429–42.

87. Hirano T, McCullough MB, Kitaoka HB, et al. Effects of foot orthoses on the work of friction of the posterior tibial tendon. Clin Biomech (Bristol, Avon) 2009;24(9):776–80.

Biomechanical Insights Afforded by Shape Modeling in the Foot and Ankle

Amy L. Lenz, PhD*, Rich J. Lisonbee, MS

KEYWORDS

- Statistical shape modeling • Morphology • Foot and ankle • Imaging
- Three-dimensional • Morphometrics • Anatomy

KEY POINTS

- Advancements in weightbearing computed tomography allows for high-resolution imaging to reconstruct bone models throughout the foot and ankle.
- Statistical shape modeling is a computational technique that can advance our understanding of complex morphology and joint interactions throughout the foot and ankle.
- The ability to computationally model and quantify three-dimensional joint relationships across multiple joints and populations allows for robust and comprehensive analyses that can influence new approaches to clinically evaluate and treat complex foot and ankle morphology.

INTRODUCTION
Nature of the Problem

Conventional radiographs are the current standard for clinically evaluating the foot and ankle but have shown substantial limitations.[1] The complex anatomy of the foot and ankle has required a variety of different two-dimensional (2D) radiographic views and clinical measurements to be clinically evaluated (eg, hindfoot, anteroposterior, lateral, and mortise views). However, these approaches lack the ability to evaluate the complex three-dimensional (3D) structures and morphometric interactions of surrounding joints or allow for visualization of the intricate ankle joint complex. Furthermore, conventional radiographs can have inherent errors due to variations in rotational positioning during image acquisition.[2] In contract, computed tomography (CT) imaging or MRI allows for more robust 3D evaluations of the patient-specific anatomy and morphology[3,4] (**Fig. 1**).

Department of Orthopaedics, University of Utah, 590 Wakara Way, Salt Lake City, UT 84108, USA
* Corresponding author.
E-mail address: amy.lenz@utah.edu

Foot Ankle Clin N Am 28 (2023) 63–76
https://doi.org/10.1016/j.fcl.2022.11.001

foot.theclinics.com

Abbreviations	
2D	Two-dimensional
3D	Three-dimensional
CT	Computed tomography
LDA	Linear discriminant analysis
OA	Osteoarthritis
PCA	Principal component analysis
SSM	Statistical shape modeling
WBCT	Weightbearing computed tomography

Weightbearing Computed Tomography Imaging

The introduction of weightbearing CT (WBCT) technology has enabled imaging of the patient in a neutral weightbearing position, offering an opportunity for more detailed analyses of the foot and ankle during loading.[4,5] Yet, many clinical studies still use individual coronal WBCT slices to conduct 2D measurements within this 3D image dataset.[4,6–11] The fast, effective, and high-resolution 3D capabilities of WBCT truly create a useful imaging tool for a variety of data analysis methods, including automatic segmentation, deep learning artificial intelligence development, and population-based statistical shape models.[12–16] As we make advancements in imaging and modeling our clinical 2D measures and metrics should advance at a faster rate to keep pace with rapid technological advancements.

BACKGROUND
What Is Statistical Shape Modeling?

Statistical shape modeling (SSM) has emerged as a computational tool to assess the 3D anatomical shape and deformity of bones throughout the body.[17–23] Although this 3D approach is promising, limitations still exist in some current applications including error-prone optimization strategies, evaluating individual bones without consideration of articulating joint relationships, and lack of clinically interpretable results from model outputs. Overall, the complexity and high variability of biological structures have contributed to the popularity of using SSMs for clinical applications. These SSMs can be used to identify group mean shapes as well as individual shape differences.

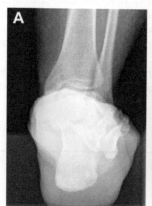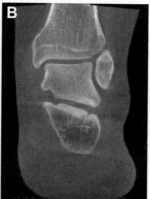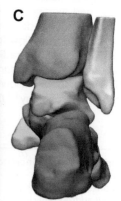

Fig. 1. Hindfoot visualization of a healthy individual with three distinct methods of assessing morphology: (*A*) Hindfoot radiograph for the Saltzman view, (*B*) WBCT coronal slice, and (*C*) 3D bone reconstruction for the tibia, fibula, talus, calcaneus, cuboid, and navicular.

There are a variety of different SSM methodologies that can identify shape differences across individuals and groups that will be discussed herein.

Not All Statistical Shape Models Are Created Equal

The evolution of SSM has led to a variety of different techniques and methods, each with their own strengths and weaknesses. A common method involves estimating the distribution of shape variation from a set of similar structures by using image registration techniques and requires correspondence mapping.[24–27] Successful registration of the correspondence across all shapes allows for mathematical investigation of the group and individual shape variations. Other methods include landmark placement done automatically or by trained raters.[21,28] A weakness of these approaches is that they limit the evaluation of shape variation to selected landmarks or features. Whereas mathematically optimizing correspondence points across the bone surfaces remove human bias and can identify shape variations that may be overlooked.

Selection of an appropriate SSM methodology to use for a particular problem is important. Just as important, is the creation of bone input models and the preprocessing techniques. Simply following a generalized SSM standard operating protocol will not result in a reliable or successful model. Conceptually, models will only be as good as the data that is input to the optimization algorithms. Inaccurate segmentation of the input bone models can lead to biased or erroneous shape variations and can be affected by the resolution of the segmented images. For example, if one direction of the 3D scan is imaged at a higher slice thickness creating segmentation pixelation or stair stepping in one axis will create poor parameterization and registration of the 3D morphology (**Fig. 2**). Conversely, overly smoothing of the bone models can result in simplified shaped bones lacking anatomical feature details (**Fig. 3**). Therefore, the key to a good SSM is to have consistency and attention to detail when creating the bone models.

CURRENT STUDIES

It is clinically well understood that different foot and ankle disease and deformities affect the underlying bony anatomy but characterizing these variations have historically been limited. Therefore, the use of SSM to characterize foot and ankle anatomy has increased in recent years. These SSM studies have sought to categorize healthy bone variation,

Talar Pixelation in Z Axis Imaging

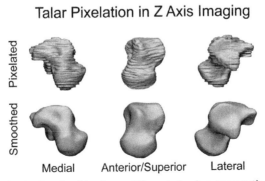

Fig. 2. The same talus is visualized in three different viewing perspectives (medial, lateral, and anterior/superior). The first row showed a native imaging resolution of 0.6 mm × 0.6 mm in the XY plane and 2 mm in the Z-axis. The 3D segmentation shows this pixelation and stair stepping in the Z-direction, whereas the second-row segmentations began with a native imaging resolution of 0.6 mm in all three planes.

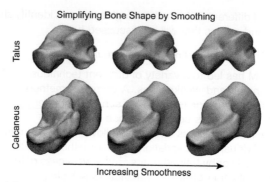

Fig. 3. Examples of the talus and calcaneus 3D reconstructions with high-quality anatomical details on the left. As the degree of smoothing increases, the level of detail decreases moving to the right. Excessive smoothing can create erroneous features that did not exist prior in some areas and remove meaningful features in other areas.

identify sex or symmetry differences, or better understand disease pathology effects on bone shape. Establishing healthy normative bone shapes is essential for understanding the foot and ankle, but what truly is "normal"? Even within healthy asymptomatic population groups, there are a variety of shape variations. These variations could be affected by any number of factors including genetics, diet, daily footwear, occupation, activity level, disease, deformity, ethnicity, among many others.[29–32]

A common element within SSM methods is the use of point/shape registration techniques. These can include but are not limited to point cloud registrations, shape registrations, or nonrigid mapping to establish correspondence,[33–37] then solving a registration algorithm resulting in an SSM (**Table 1**). The solution and evaluation of these registration algorithms vary, and each combination has their own strengths and weaknesses. In short there is a variety of different methods to develop and validate an SSM. Although there may be common themes, each method has an impact that may result in no two methodologies yielding an identical statistical model from the same data set.

Spherical Harmonics

Work by Melinska and colleagues[22,23] used spherical harmonics to create statistical models to characterize the mean shape of the calcaneus, cuboid, navicular, and talus bones. The spherical harmonics description is computed from the mesh and its spherical parametrizations are then aligned to establish correspondence across all surfaces.[38] This method required manual selected seed points for the extraction of the bone contours and manual marked bone surfaces to position features. Whenever manual selection is required, it introduces bias that may affect the resulting SSM, which was acknowledged as a possible hindrance within their studies, then suggesting that shape registration methods could be used. Although this work was able to produce statistical models, their results qualitatively appeared more ellipsoidal than expected, and used correlations of spherical harmonic coefficients to compare shape variation.

Gaussian Processes

There are a few studies that have created statistical models using Gaussian processes fit to the data. This process computes a low-rank approximation using the Nyström method and then formulates the registration as a parametric optimization problem.[39] Studies that have cited this methodology include modeling talar bone shape variations

Table 1
Summary of articles published on statistical shape modeling (SSM) with reported topics, anatomical models of interest, imaging source for input bone reconstructions, and SSM methods

Topic	Model(s)	Imaging	SSM Methods	Citation
Cross-sectional OA	Hindfoot	Radiographs	Landmark placement[47]	Nelson et al.[21] 2017
Functional segments of Foot	Foot segments	MRI (1 mm³)	Point cloud registration	Grant et al.[33] 2020
Sex differences	Tibia, talus, and calcaneus	CT (0.59 mm³ and 0.72 mm³)	Automatic landmark matching algorithm[54]	Gabrielli et al.[34] 2020
Pediatric clubfoot	Talus	MRI (0.6–4 mm³)	Shape registration[35]	Feng et al.[35] 2021
Tibia-fibula complex	Tibia and fibula	CT (0.488 × 0.488 × 0.625 mm³)	Coherent point drift[27]	Bruce et al.[37] 2020
Syndesmotic ankle lesions	Tibia and fibula	CT (0.6 mm³)	Point surface matching[55]	Peiffer et al.[36] 2022
Calcaneus average shape	Calcaneus	CT	Spherical harmonics[56]	Melinska et al.[23] 2015
Cuboid, navicular, and talus average shape (Atlas)	Cuboid, navicular, and talus	CT	Spherical harmonics[56]	Melinska et al.[22] 2017
Ankle impingement	Talus	CT (0.98 × 0.98 × 0.70 mm³ control, 0.98 × 0.98 × 0.45 mm³ impingement)	Gaussian process[39]	Arbab et al.[40] 2022
Symmetry and gissane measurements	Calcaneus	CT	Gaussian process[39]	Schmutz et al.[41] 2021
Talar prostheses	Talus	CT (0.36 × 0.36 mm²)	Gaussian process[39]	Vafaeian et al.[57] 2022
Symmetry	Tibia, fibula, talus, and calcaneus	CT (0.63 × 0.63 × 0.70 mm³ and 0.98 × 0.98 × 0.70 mm³)	Parallel groupwise registration[26]	Tümer et al.[42] 2019
Chronic ankle instability	Talus and calcaneus	CT (0.3 × 0.3 × 0.3 mm³ and 0.7 × 0.5 × 0.5 mm³)	Parallel groupwise registration[26]	Tümer et al.[43] 2019
Talus average shape	Talus	CT (0.6 mm³)	Parallel groupwise registration[26]	Liu et al.[44] 2020

(continued on next page)

Table 1
(continued)

Topic	Model(s)	Imaging	SSM Methods	Citation
Tibia, fibula, and talus mean shape	Tibia, fibula, and talus	WBCT (0.4 mm³)	Entropy-based particle system[25,53]	Lenz et al.[16] 2021
Talus and calcaneus mean shape	Talus and calcaneus	WBCT (0.4 mm³)	Entropy-based particle system[25,53]	Krähenbühl et al.[15] 2020
Multi-bone model of the subtalar, talonavicular, and calcaneocuboid joints	Talus, calcaneus, navicular, and cuboid	WBCT (0.4 mm³)	Entropy-based particle system[25,53]	Peterson et al.[45] 2022
Foot morphology	26 bones	MRI (0.5 mm³)	Entropy-based particle system[25,53]	Welshman et al.[46] 2021

in patient populations with ankle impingement,[40] and morphological variability in calcaneal shape relating to Gissane's crucial angle.[41]

Parallel Groupwise Registration

Another method for developing an SSM is fitting an evolving mean shape to each of the shapes and performing point registration.[26] A benefit of using this algorithm is it reduces the associated expensive computational and memory costs involved when calculating point cloud registration algorithms. This allows for a higher number of shapes to be included in the model development with similar hardware. Some studies that have used this methodology within the foot and ankle have investigated shape variations and symmetry of the hindfoot,[42] shape differences of the subtalar bones in patient groups with chronic ankle instability,[43] and average shape of the talus for talar implant designs.[44]

Particle-Based Entropy System

The last SSM method we will discuss constructs statistical models from correspondence particles distributed across the shape surfaces via energy functions.[25] This method utilizes a point-based sampling of the shapes while simultaneously maximizing both the geometric accuracy and the statistical simplicity of the model. Accomplished by optimizing sample positions by gradient descent of an energy function balancing the negative entropy of the distribution of each shape with the positive entropy of the ensemble of shapes. A weakness of this strategy is that it requires parameter tuning to generate valuable correspondence models. Work by the authors has employed this methodology to create statistical models of the bones of the subtalar joint,[15] talocrural joint,[16] and talonavicular/calcaneocuboid joints.[45] With this method readily available in a free public software platform (ShapeWorks), others have used this method recently to model multi-domain shapes encompassing more of the foot and ankle.[46] All these models have reported variations of morphology seen in healthy populations to establish statistical distributions of the anatomy.

MODEL EVALUATION
Principal Component Analysis

When evaluating the results from an SSM, a principal component analysis (PCA) is typically performed.[47] A PCA decomposes a multivariate data set into its mean and corresponding covariance matrix. The eigenvectors from this covariance matrix are referred to as the principal components and the eigenvalues indicate the relative importance of those components. This analysis results in principal shape variations that can be used to compare shape modes of variations and describe shape differences within a population. The PCA modes containing significant variation are typically determined using parallel analysis.[48]

An example of a multi-domain statistical model's PCA results is shown (**Fig. 4**). This model was created from the talus, navicular, calcaneus, and cuboid from 27 asymptomatic individuals (ShapeWorks) and illustrates the first two modes of variation and their respective ±2 standard deviations of shape.[45] Modes of variation were identified then rank ordered from highest to lowest eigenvalues from the principal components with key modes determined via a parallel analysis. Significant modes of variation may contain key features or shape variations that are clinically relevant. For example, mode 1 characterizes the overall size variation across the population, indicating the interplay of relative size of these four peritalar bones across the population of patients with a reported height of 169.4 ± 6.4 cm. Features from the second mode, indicated by

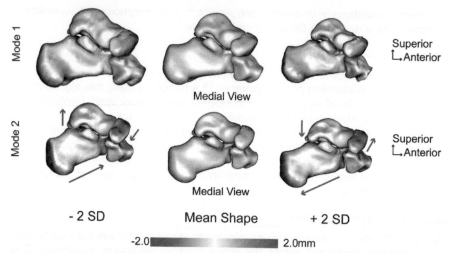

Fig. 4. First and second modes of variation of the multi-domain model consisting of the talus, calcaneus, navicular and cuboid. The shape variation from these modes is shown by point-to-mesh surface distances (CloudCompare). Surfaces expanding outward of the mean shape surface are highlighted in red and surfaces reducing into the surface of the mean shape are highlighted in blue. Key observed variations are indicated by an arrow.

red arrows, show that as the calcaneus shortens the calcaneus height increases and conversely as the calcaneus lengthens the calcaneus height shortens. Observations from the talonavicular and calcaneocuboid joints show a more superior alignment of the navicular and cuboid with a longer calcaneus, changing the midfoot articulation relative to the calcaneal pitch.

Linear Discriminant Analysis

A linear discriminant analysis (LDA) can also be conducted to characterize various shapes between different populations (**Fig. 5**). In this example, two groups of patients

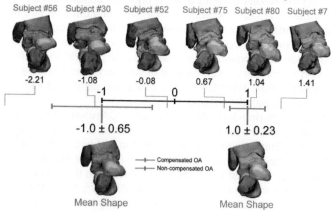

Fig. 5. Linear discriminant model displaying shape scores for bone alignment and morphology between two groups with ankle osteoarthritis (OA): non-compensated (*orange*) and compensated (*blue*).

with osteoarthritis (OA) are classified along a normalized scale from -1 to 1, with the non-compensated OA group mean classified at -1 and the compensated OA group classified at 1. The LDA generates shape scores for each patient's bone across the normalized scale that can then be displayed relative to the mean group shapes. These shape scores could be used in the assessment of patient pathology or deformity severity. In this example notice that the standard deviations of the two mean groups shown below the normalized scale are not overlapping and the variability in the compensated OA group is very tight. This indicates that the morphology and alignment represented in the overall shape score of these two groups are statistically different from one another, when these shape scores were compared with a t-test ($P<.05$). Next, six representative patients are visualized above the normalized scale with their patient-specific shape scores across the spectrum. Clinically we can observe that the most severe patient with non-compensated OA has a more vertically aligned talonavicular and calcaneocuboid joints with a greater distance from the distal end of the fibula to the talus. This results in an overall varus hindfoot alignment. On the opposite spectrum of deformity, the most severe patient with compensated OA shows a more neutral alignment of the hindfoot with a varus tibiotalar joint and a valgus subtalar joint to achieve this overall aligned hindfoot. Consequently, the talonavicular and calcaneocuboid joints are more typically aligned and the distance between the fibula and the talus is reduced.

Quantitative Evaluation Metrics—Compactness, Generalization, and Specificity

Quantitative metrics of compactness, generalization, and specificity can be used to assess the shape-correspondence performance with respect to the model's construction and optimization.[49-51] These measures collectively evaluate the quality of the shape model from correspondence particles and are defined as a function of the number of modes, under the assumption that the shape model is built using a PCA.

Compactness is the quantitative evaluation of the amount of variance in the underlying shape model. Two approaches for compactness are commonly computed: (1) according to the number of components that account for 95% of the accumulated variance, or (2) as the sum of the eigenvalues for a given subspace up to the total number of modes reported. A higher compactness measure is better because it can explain the shape with fewer modes of variation.

Generalization is defined as the ability of the shape model to accurately represent unseen shapes of the structure model that are outside of the data set. It is quantified as an approximation error calculated by the means of a leave-one-out cross-validation approach. The approximation error is then calculated in terms of Euclidean distance between the held-out shape instance and the closest training sample. For two models built using the same training data, the model with a lower generalization error indicates a better shape model that can represent structures not included in the data set.

Specificity quantifies the ability of the shape model to generate new probable instances of the shapes by constraining the variability in the shape space using the learned population-specific shape statistics and comparing them to structures in the training data set. Specificity generally increases with the number of modes considered. A model with a lower specificity indicates that the model is more specific and can generate probable instances from that subspace.

DISCUSSION

With any statistical model there is bound to be a wide variety of shape variation. As scientists and engineers, we can characterize anatomical shape variations in subsets of the population ad nauseam, but it is critical to consider the clinical perspective in our findings from SSM and how they impact patient care and inform our understanding.

So how can we use SSM as a clinical tool to help improve treatment or guide preventative care? Thanks to deep learning artificial intelligence development and advancements in automatic segmentation, generating patient-specific bone models can now be done as part of daily clinical practice.[52] Ideally these patient-specific bone models could then be evaluated against a vetted SSM to help identify risk factors for disease or deformity progression. An obstacle with SSM includes a need for larger data sets. To effectively identify potential morphometric risk factors or characterize trends in morphology we need appropriately large sets of data from which to draw anatomical conclusions. As imaging processing techniques become faster, better quality, and more reliable, readily obtaining bone models of large study cohorts is a near reality. Ideally, to characterize bone morphology across the human spectrum we need to image and collect data across the human spectrum. This goal requires an enormous amount of effort, both financially and computationally. For translational research we need clinician buy in and more open-source image data sets to better capture and model the human spectrum.

But a lack of all current SSM approaches is the optimized outputs are still a mathematical description of shape. Therefore, most papers will report the eigenvalue variance and significant explanation of variance, but not include what the interpretation is of these values. For the papers that do describe anatomical features found in modes of variation, this was performed manually using detailed knowledge of anatomical landmarks. The future of SSM could be integrating in musculoskeletal radiologist and/or orthopedic surgeon impression lists into models to increase the predictability of significant features or interpretation of the modes of variation seen from SSMs. Therefore, at this time, SSMs are only as good as their clinical interpretation, making collaboration with clinicians to be paramount for excelling in these research efforts.

As noted herein, not all SSM approaches are created equally based on varying computational techniques that may or may not require manual selection of landmarks that can introduce human bias. In general, model optimizations should be carefully considered and known limitations of the model should be acknowledged before using any computational approach. However, methods that provide unbiased evaluation of the full 3D bone surface will be most beneficial to characterizing shape variations and even joint relationships in a multi-bone (ie, multi-domain) model. With advancing computational models, and by reporting the quality of the model or even providing open-source repositories of finalized models, we can grow as a field by peer-verification and consistent computational methods. At the end of the day, to grow the use of SSM in the field of foot and ankle, we should encourage collaborative big-data initiatives to truly characterize foot and ankle morphology across various pathologies and deformities.

Future Directions

With a relatively minimal set of literature focusing on foot and ankle morphology using SSM, the future of this field has room for tremendous growth. First, a worldwide initiative to create an open-source atlas of foot and ankle morphology across the spectrum of deformities and pathologies could serve as a pivotal adoption of SSM. Through this atlas, the field could move away from performing 2D clinical measurements and instead use 3D measurements from SSM to identify abnormal anatomy. Future work developing an SSM of coupled structures throughout the foot and ankle, or multi-domain models, could also describe relationships between structures, such as articulating relationships between bones and their alignment to identify not only bone level abnormalities but coupled deformities.[53] This approach could be applied to the whole WBCT scan of a new patient and incorporated into the already optimized SSM-generated atlas to identify key clinical features. SSM could also be applied to longitudinal datasets of WBCTs to monitor changes overtime to understand disease progression, structural development, or fracture healing, to name a few. As computational efficiencies are advancing the field of image processing, the future use of SSM for numerous clinical applications is becoming a reality.

SUMMARY

The complex nature of foot and ankle joint morphology has primarily been analyzed from 2D measurements on clinical conventional radiographs. The advent of WBCT has opened a new era of possibilities for 3D modeling. 3D volumetric image data are available with this novel imaging modality, yet research and clinical evaluation is still primarily limited to 2D slice measurements. SSM has emerged as a computational tool to assess the 3D anatomical shape and deformity of bones. Improved SSM optimization methods remove human bias and even have the ability to model combined joint-level analyses. But the widespread use of SSM is still limited in the field. Future work can expand the use of SSM to characterize multiple patient cohorts across the spectrum of foot and ankle diagnoses. With the establishment of a morphology atlas, foot and ankle surgeons can use these 3D tools to visualize patient morphology for improved treatment planning, diagnosis, and longitudinal tracking of disease progression in groundbreaking ways that were previously not possible.

CLINICS CARE POINTS

- When visually assessing statistical shape modeling results, it is important to collaborate with an interdisciplinary team to identify meaningful conclusions driven by clinical hypotheses.

- With the high-resolution volumetric data available in weightbearing computed tomography scans, clinicians should be cautioned to not only use single slice two-dimensional measurements and are advised to also consider using three-dimensional representations of the structures for clinical evaluations and surgical decision making.

- Clinical measurements and metrics need to advance with new innovative technologies. Current clinical measures may be limited in their ability to accurately assess foot and ankle disease and disorders.

DISCLOSURE

The National Institutes of Health supported this work under grant number NIAMS-K01AR080221.

REFERENCES

1. Lintz F, de Cesar Netto C, Barg A, et al. Weight-bearing cone beam CT scans in the foot and ankle. EFORT Open Rev 2018;3(5):278–86.
2. Krahenbuhl N, Lenz AL, Lisonbee R, et al. Imaging of the subtalar joint: a novel approach to an old problem. J Orthop Res 2019. https://doi.org/10.1002/jor.24220.
3. Hayes A, Tochigi Y, Saltzman CL. Ankle morphometry on 3D-CT images. Iowa Orthopaedic J 2006;26:1–4.

4. Barg A, Bailey T, Richter M, et al. Weightbearing computed tomography of the foot and ankle: emerging technology topical review. Foot Ankle Int 2018;39(3): 376–86.

5. Krähenbühl N, Horn-Lang T, Hintermann B, et al. The subtalar joint. EFORT Open Rev 2017;2(7):309–16.

6. Krahenbuhl N, Siegler L, Deforth M, et al. Subtalar joint alignment in ankle osteoarthritis. Foot Ankle Surg 2017. https://doi.org/10.1016/j.fas.2017.10.004.

7. Krahenbuhl N, Tschuck M, Bolliger L, et al. Orientation of the Subtalar Joint: Measurement and Reliability Using Weightbearing CT Scans. Foot Ankle Int 2016; 37(1):109–14.

8. Cody EA, Williamson ER, Burket JC, et al. Correlation of talar anatomy and subtalar joint alignment on weightbearing computed tomography with radiographic flatfoot parameters. Foot Ankle Int 2016. https://doi.org/10.1177/1071100716646629.

9. Probasco W, Haleem AM, Yu J, et al. Assessment of coronal plane subtalar joint alignment in peritalar subluxation via weight-bearing multiplanar imaging. Foot Ankle Int 2014. https://doi.org/10.1177/1071100714557861.

10. Colin F, Horn Lang T, Zwicky L, et al. Subtalar joint configuration on weightbearing CT scan. Foot Ankle Int 2014;35(10):1057–62.

11. Apostle KL, Coleman NW, Sangeorzan BJ. Subtalar joint axis in patients with symptomatic peritalar subluxation compared to normal controls. Foot Ankle Int 2014;35(11):1153–8.

12. Day J, De Cesar Netto C, Richter M, et al. Evaluation of a weightbearing CT artificial intelligence-based automatic measurement for the M1-M2 intermetatarsal angle in hallux valgus. Foot Ankle Int 2021;42(11):1502–9.

13. Kvarda P, Heisler L, Krähenbühl N, et al. 3D Assessment in Posttraumatic Ankle Osteoarthritis. Foot Ankle Int 2021;42(2):200–14.

14. Krähenbühl N, Kvarda P, Susdorf R, et al. Assessment of progressive collapsing foot deformity using semiautomated 3D measurements derived from weightbearing CT scans. Foot Ankle Int 2021. https://doi.org/10.1177/10711007211049754. 107110072110497.

15. Krähenbühl N, Lenz AL, Lisonbee RJ, et al. Morphologic analysis of the subtalar joint using statistical shape modeling. J Orthopaedic Res 2020;38(12):2625–33.

16. Lenz AL, Krähenbühl N, Peterson AC, et al. Statistical shape modeling of the talocrural joint using a hybrid multi-articulation joint approach. Scientific Rep 2021; 11(1). https://doi.org/10.1038/s41598-021-86567-7.

17. Agricola R, Leyland KM, Bierma-Zeinstra SM, et al. Validation of statistical shape modelling to predict hip osteoarthritis in females: data from two prospective cohort studies (Cohort Hip and Cohort Knee and Chingford). Rheumatology (Oxford, England) 2015;54(11):2033–41.

18. Atkins PR, Elhabian SY, Agrawal P, et al. Quantitative comparison of cortical bone thickness using correspondence-based shape modeling in patients with cam femoroacetabular impingement. J Orthop Res 2016. https://doi.org/10.1002/jor.23468.

19. Harris MD, Datar M, Whitaker RT, et al. Statistical shape modeling of cam femoroacetabular impingement. J Orthop Res 2013;31(10):1620–6.

20. Ma J, Wang A, Lin F, et al. A novel robust kernel principal component analysis for nonlinear statistical shape modeling from erroneous data. Comput Med Imaging Graphics 2019;77:101638.

21. Nelson AE, Golightly YM, Lateef S, et al. Cross-sectional associations between variations in ankle shape by statistical shape modeling, injury history, and race: the Johnston County Osteoarthritis Project. J Foot Ankle Res 2017;10:34.

22. Melinska AU, Romaszkiewicz P, Wagel J, et al. Statistical shape models of cuboid, navicular and talus bones. J Foot Ankle Res 2017;10:6.

23. Melinska AU, Romaszkiewicz P, Wagel J, et al. Statistical, morphometric, anatomical shape model (atlas) of calcaneus. PLoS One 2015;10(8):e0134603.

24. Ambellan F, Lamecker H, von Tycowicz C, et al. Statistical shape models: understanding and mastering variation in anatomy. Adv Exp Med Biol 2019;1156: 67–84.

25. Cates J, Fletcher PT, Styner M, et al. Shape modeling and analysis with entropy-based particle systems. Inf Process Med Imaging 2007;20:333–45.

26. Van De Giessen M, Vos FM, Grimbergen CA, et al. An efficient and robust algorithm for parallel groupwise registration of bone surfaces. Berlin, Germany: Springer Berlin Heidelberg; 2012. p. 164–71.

27. Myronenko A, Xubo S. Point set registration: coherent point drift. IEEE Trans Pattern Anal Machine Intelligence 2010;32(12):2262–75.

28. Qiang M, Chen Y, Zhang K, et al. Measurement of three-dimensional morphological characteristics of the calcaneus using CT image post-processing. J Foot Ankle Res 2014;7(1):19.

29. Tasnim N, Schmitt D, Zeininger A. Effects of human variation on foot and ankle pain in rural Madagascar. Am J Phys Anthropol 2021;176(2):308–20.

30. Zhao X, Tsujimoto T, Kim B, et al. Characteristics of foot morphology and their relationship to gender, age, body mass index and bilateral asymmetry in Japanese adults. J Back Musculoskelet Rehabil 2017;30(3):527–35.

31. Barisch-Fritz B, Schmeltzpfenning T, Plank C, et al. Foot deformation during walking: differences between static and dynamic 3D foot morphology in developing feet. Ergonomics 2014;57(6):921–33.

32. Yurt Y, Sener G, Yakut Y. Footwear suitability in Turkish preschool-aged children. Prosthetics and Orthotics International 2014;38(3):224–31.

33. Grant TM, Diamond LE, Pizzolato C, et al. Development and validation of statistical shape models of the primary functional bone segments of the foot. Peer J 2020;8:e8397. https://doi.org/10.7717/peerj.8397.

34. Gabrielli AS, Gale T, Hogan M, et al. Bilateral Symmetry, Sex Differences, and Primary Shape Factors in Ankle and Hindfoot Bone Morphology. Foot & Ankle Orthopaedics 2020;5(1). https://doi.org/10.1177/2473011420908796. 247301142090879.

35. Feng Y, Bishop A, Farley D, et al. Statistical shape modelling to analyse the talus in paediatric clubfoot. Proc Inst Mech Eng H: J Eng Med 2021;235(8):849–60.

36. Peiffer M, Burssens A, De Mits S, et al. Statistical shape model-based tibiofibular assessment of syndesmotic ankle lesions using weight-bearing CT. J Orthopaedic Res 2022. https://doi.org/10.1002/jor.25318.

37. Bruce OL, Baggaley M, Welte L, et al. A statistical shape model of the tibia-fibula complex: sexual dimorphism and effects of age on reconstruction accuracy from anatomical landmarks. Computer Methods Biomech Biomed Eng 2022;25(8): 875–86.

38. Styner M, Oguz I, Xu S, et al. Framework for the statistical shape analysis of brain structures using SPHARM-PDM. Insight J 2006;1071:242–50.

39. Lüthi M, Jud C, Vetter T. A unified approach to shape model fitting and non-rigid registration. Cham, Switzerland: Springer International Publishing; 2013. p. 66–73.

40. Arbabi S, Seevinck P, Weinans H, et al. Statistical shape model of the talus bone morphology: A comparison between impinged and nonimpinged ankles. J Orthopaedic Res 2022. https://doi.org/10.1002/jor.25328.

41. Schmutz B, Lüthi M, Schmutz-Leong YK, et al. Morphological analysis of Gissane's angle utilising a statistical shape model of the calcaneus. Arch Orthopaedic Trauma Surg 2021;141(6):937–45.

42. Tümer N, Arbabi V, Gielis WP, et al. Three-dimensional analysis of shape variations and symmetry of the fibula, tibia, calcaneus and talus. J Anat 2019; 234(1):132–44.

43. Tümer N, Vuurberg G, Blankevoort L, et al. Typical shape differences in the subtalar joint bones between subjects with chronic ankle instability and controls. J Orthopaedic Res 2019;37(9):1892–902.

44. Liu T, Jomha NM, Adeeb S, et al. Investigation of the Average Shape and Principal Variations of the Human Talus Bone Using Statistic Shape Model. Original Research. Front Bioeng Biotechnol 2020;8. https://doi.org/10.3389/fbioe.2020.00656.

45. Peterson AC, Lisonbee RJ, Krähenbühl N, et al. Multi-Level Multi-Domain Statistical Shape Model of the Subtalar, Talonavicular, and Calcaneocuboid Joints. Front Bioeng Biotechnol 2022;10:1–17.

46. Welshman ZMS. A novel analytical pipeline quantifying variance in foot morphology and function using statistical shape modelling and a 26-segment foot model. UK: University of Leeds; 2021.

47. Cootes TF, Taylor CJ, Cooper DH, et al. Training models of shape from sets of examples. London, UK: Springer; 1992. p. 9–18.

48. Horn JL. A rationale and test for the number of factors in factor analysis. Psychometrika 1965;30(2):179–85.

49. Wang J, Shi C. Automatic construction of statistical shape models using deformable simplex meshes with vector field convolution energy. Biomed Eng Online 2017;16(1):49.

50. Davies RH. Learning shape: optimal models for analysing natural variability. Manchester, UK: The University of Manchester; 2002.

51. Styner MA, Rajamani KT, Nolte LP, et al. Evaluation of 3D correspondence methods for model building. Information processing in medical imaging : Proceedings of the Conference. Jul 2003;18:63-75. doi:

52. Ortolani M, Leardini A, Pavani C, et al. Angular and linear measurements of adult flexible flatfoot via weight-bearing CT scans and 3D bone reconstruction tools. Scientific Rep 2021;11(1):16139.

53. Cates J, Fletcher PT, Styner M, et al. Particle-based shape analysis of multi-object complexes. Med Image Comput Comput Assist Interv 2008;11(Pt 1):477–85.

54. Lansdown DA, Pedoia V, Zaid M, et al. Variations in knee kinematics After ACL injury and after reconstruction are correlated with bone shape differences. Clin Orthop Relat Res 2017;475(10):2427–35.

55. Audenaert EA, Pattyn C, Steenackers G, et al. Statistical shape modeling of skeletal anatomy for sex discrimination: their training size, sexual dimorphism, and asymmetry. original research. Front Bioeng Biotechnol 2019;7. https://doi.org/10.3389/fbioe.2019.00302.

56. Iskander DR. Modeling videokeratoscopic height data with spherical harmonics. Optom Vis Sci 2009;86(5):542–7.

57. Vafaeian B, Riahi HT, Amoushahi H, et al. A feature-based statistical shape model for geometric analysis of the human talus and development of universal talar prostheses. J Anat 2022;240(2):305–22.

Biomechanical Sequelae of Syndesmosis Injury and Repair

Jennifer A. Nichols, PhD[a,b,]*, Chloe Baratta, BS[a],
Christopher W. Reb, DO[c]

KEYWORDS

- Tibiofibular joint • Fibula • Kinematics • Kinetics • High ankle sprain • Ligament
- Contact mechanics • Fixation

KEY POINTS

- Fibular motion is an essential component of ankle joint function. Tibiofibular movement in the ankle syndesmosis provides stability and shock absorption while facilitating load transfer from the femur through the talocrural articulations.
- Arthrokinematics and loading patterns across the foot and ankle change in the presence of syndesmosis injury and repair. However, the clinical consequences of these changes are poorly understood.
- Subject-specific factors, such as bone morphology, injury pattern, injury severity, and fixation approach, impact pre- and postoperative fibula mechanics.
- An ideal fixation construct and/or surgical technique capable of matching fibula mechanics between intact and repaired syndesmoses has not yet been identified.
- Fully understanding the relationship between fibular mechanics and outcomes requires in vivo data evaluating mechanics and outcomes in a single, patient cohort.

INTRODUCTION

The importance of the fibula is often overlooked. For example, when sacrificing the fibula to provide autologous bone grafts or when leaving the fibula out of analyses of ankle biomechanics, we choose to prioritize other clinical concerns above the functional role of the fibula. Yet, the human fibula is critically important to lower limb mechanics. As part of only two orders in the animal kingdom with mobile fibulae (namely,

Disclosure: The authors have no commercial or financial conflicts of interest to disclose.
[a] J. Crayton Pruitt Family Department of Biomedical Engineering, University of Florida, 1275 Center Drive, Gainesville, FL 32611, USA; [b] Department of Orthopaedic Surgery & Sports Medicine, University of Florida, 3450 Hull Road, Gainesville, FL, 32607, USA; [c] Orthopaedics, Veterans Health Administration North Florida / South Georgia Health System, Malcolm Randall VA Medical Center, 1601 SW Archer Road, Gainesville, FL, 32608, USA
* Corresponding author. P.O. Box 116131, Gainesville, FL 32611.
E-mail address: jnichols@bme.ufl.edu

Foot Ankle Clin N Am 28 (2023) 77–98
https://doi.org/10.1016/j.fcl.2022.10.004
1083-7515/23/© 2022 Elsevier Inc. All rights reserved.

foot.theclinics.com

Primates and Carnivora, in which cats and bears have mobile fibulae),[1] humans rely on their fibulae for ankle joint stability and load transfer.

Syndesmosis injuries disrupt fibula function by damaging the integrity of the tibiofibular ligaments. Both conservative and surgical treatment of syndesmosis injuries aim to restore tibiofibular mechanics. However, even following surgery, syndesmosis injuries impart a large negative effect on functional outcomes.[2] Thus, fibula dysfunction (i.e., altered mechanics) persists following treatment.

The goal of this review is to describe fibula mechanics in the context of syndesmosis injury and repair. A deep understanding of fibula biomechanics has the potential to inform clinical management of the ankle syndesmosis and inspire future work into effectively minimizing fibula dysfunction. We divide the review into three main sections describing the intact ankle, syndesmosis injury, and syndesmosis repair. Each section begins with a brief primer on the clinical context. This is followed by an in-depth summary of fibular mechanics, which includes discussion of kinematics (the study of motion) and kinetics (the study of forces that cause motion). We conclude with a discussion of clinical considerations for managing syndesmosis injuries and how those considerations relate to current gaps in knowledge and potential areas for future research.

INTACT ANKLE
Anatomy of the Healthy Syndesmosis

The distal tibiofibular syndesmosis, or ankle syndesmosis, is a fibrous joint consisting of the incisura tibialis, the lateral malleolus of the fibula, and the four strong ligamentous connections between them (**Fig. 1**; see Hermans and colleagues[3] for detailed review). The anterior inferior tibiofibular ligament (AITFL), posterior inferior tibiofibular ligament (PITFL), and fibrocartilaginous inferior transverse ligaments are specialized for fibula constraint.[4] The interosseous ligament is contiguous with the interosseous membrane. Although these anatomic elements are consistently present, considerable morphologic variation is found between individuals[5–7] and between sides of the same individual.[8,9]

Healthy Fibular Motion

The ankle bones form an interconnected, kinematic chain, meaning motion of the fibula, tibia, and talus are interdependent. Early cadaveric studies note this interdependence by highlighting the fibula's role in ankle stability. For example, during foot-floor contact, the fibula laterally stabilizes the ankle mortise while simultaneously providing

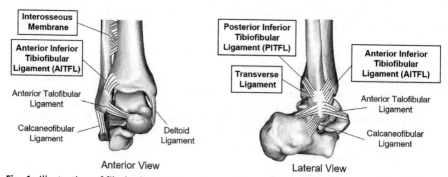

Anterior View   Lateral View

Fig. 1. Illustration of fibular ligament anatomy. Ligaments comprising the ankle syndesmosis are highlighted in bold and placed in boxes.

shock absorption.[10] Studies of this era also hint at the small, but complex motions experienced by the fibula.[11–16]

In a modern cadaveric study, Leardini and colleagues[17] confirmed the fibula exhibits small, tri-planar rotations during passive ankle motion. Subsequent cadaveric studies indicate the fibula also translates (e.g.,[18–20]). For example, in a recent study that measured micro-motion of the syndesmosis under various loading conditions and postures, Hu and colleagues[20] found that when the syndesmosis is placed under axial load and the ankle is dorsiflexed, the distal fibula moves laterally and posteriorly while also externally rotating, whereas when the ankle is plantarflexed, the distal fibula translates medially and anteriorly while internally rotating. Thus, the fibula rotates and translates, but the direction and magnitude of this motion varies with posture and loading.

A variety of *in vivo* methods, including motion capture, marker-based Roentegen stereophotogrammetric analysis (RSA), weight-bearing computed tomography (WBCT), 4D computed tomography (4D CT), and bi-plane fluoroscopy, have also been used to measure fibular motion.[14,15,21–34] These studies corroborate cadaveric findings by consistently demonstrating that the magnitude of fibula rotation and translation is small, and the direction of that motion varies with the task (**Table 1**). For example, in a study of six adult males that measured the motion of the foot and ankle using bone pins, Lundgren and colleagues[25] reported fibula rotational range of motion during barefoot walking at a self-selected speed as 4.7° (range 2.8° to 7.1°), 3.3° (range 2.0° to 4.9°), and 3.5° (range 2.4° to 5.7°) in the sagittal, coronal, and transverse planes, respectively. The magnitudes reported by other RSA studies[14,15,21,24] as well as WBCT and 4D CT studies,[26–29,31] which measure fibula motion between serially imaged static postures, are generally smaller than those reported by Lundgren and colleagues.[25]

Interestingly, the magnitude of fibula motion reported by bi-plane fluoroscopy studies is similar to or larger than those reported by Lundgren and colleagues.[25] In a study of sixteen adults, Wang and colleagues[32] reported that during the stance phase of gait the average tibiofibular rotational range of motion is 2.98°, 5.94°, and 5.99° in the sagittal, coronal, and transverse planes, respectively, and the average translational range of motion is 2.63 mm (medial-lateral), 3.86 mm (anterior–posterior), and 4.12 mm (superior–inferior). Comparatively, in a study of two adult females, Pitcairn and colleagues[33] reported tibiofibular range of motion across seven activities to be as high as 4.0°, 4.0°, and 14.3° in the sagittal, coronal, and transverse planes, respectively; this study did not report translations. In a study of six young, athletic adults, Hogg-Cornejo and colleagues[34] reported tibiofibular motion across four activities to be slightly lower, with reported maximums of 1.7°, 1.7°, and 9.4° in the sagittal, coronal, and transverse planes, respectively; translations were as high as 1.7 mm (medial-lateral), 2.2 mm (anterior–posterior), and 2.5 mm (superior–inferior). Because the tasks reported in these bi-plane fluoroscopy studies do not overlap, direct quantitative comparisons are not possible. In addition, to the best of our knowledge, despite a growing number of bi-plane fluoroscopy studies of the ankle, these are the only three to include fibular motion.

Of contextual importance to this discussion, *in vivo* studies show that differences in hip and knee posture influence the position of the fibula.[35,36] Because the full lower limb is rarely included in cadaver studies of the ankle, and posture across the whole lower limb is rarely reported in *in vivo* studies, it is impossible to discern to what extent differences in posture contribute to differences in reported results. Studies also include different quantities of muscle activity (from no activity in cadaver studies to variable levels of activity in quasi-static and dynamic tasks), which directly influences

Table 1
Healthy fibular range of motion reported by in vivo studies[a]

Study	n	Task	Rotational Range of Motion (Degrees)			Translational Range of Motion (mm)		
			Sagittal Plane (Dorsiflexion–Plantarflexion)	Coronal Plane (Eversion–Inversion)	Transverse Plane (External/Internal Rotation)	Sagittal Plane (Anterior–Posterior)	Coronal Plane (Medial–Lateral)	Transverse Plane (Superior–Inferior)
RSA								
Kärrholm et al. (1985)[21]	9	Ankle flexion–extension	–	–	–	0.5–2.4		
Ahl et al. (1987).[22]	7	Flexion–extension	–	–	0.0 ± 1.0	0.2 ± 0.4	–0.7 ± 0.3	0.1 ± 0.2
		Pronation–supination	–	–	0.0 ± 0.6	0.0 ± 0.2	0.0 ± 0.3	0.0 ± 0.1
Lundberg et al. (1989)[14]	8	Flexion–extension	<1	<1	<1	1	1	<0.1
Svensson et al. (1989)[15]	8	Flexion–extension	0.4	1.1	1.5	1.04	1.03	<0.1
		Pronation–supination	0.3	0.2	0.5	0.29	0.08	0.1
		Internal–external rotation	<0.6	<0.6	<0.6	<0.7	<0.7	<0.7
Beumer et al. (2003)[23,b]	11	Weight-bearing	0.00 [–0.92–0.80]	0.01 [–0.68–0.66]	0.03 [–1.28–1.18]	–0.10 [–0.96–0.28]	–0.02 [–0.41–0.44]	0.00 [–0.37–0.30]
		External rotation weight-bearing	0.12 [0.94–1.47]	–0.27 [–0.97–0.41]	–0.02 [–1.38–1.02]	–0.46 [–1.98–0.56]	0.11 [–0.19–0.63]	–0.12 [–0.59–0.23]
		External rotation stress (supine)	0.06 [–0.49–0.76]	1.20 [0.21–2.10]	–3.85 [–5.33–1.89]	–1.87 [–3.08–0.95]	1.48 [–0.06–2.52]	0.22 [–0.14–0.56]

	n							
Bone Pins								
Arndt et al. (2007)[24]	4	Running	3.3 ± 2.4	2.3 ± 0.9	1.6 ± 0.3	—	—	—
Lundgren et al. (2008)[25]	6	Walking	4.7 ± 1.6	3.3 ± 1.2	3.5 ± 1.2	—	—	—
WBCT								
Lepojärvi et al. (2016)[26]	32	Internal–external rotation	—	—	3.2 ± 2.8	1.5 ± 0.9	—	—
Hoogervorst et al. (2019)[27]	9	Weight-bearing	—	—	0.5 [−2.2–1.2]	0.2 [−0.9–0.5]	0.3 [−0.6–0.1]	—
Malhotra et al. (2019)[28,c]	26	Weight-bearing	—	—	—	0.19	0.6	—
4D CT								
Jend et al. (1985)[29]	25	Flexion–extension	—	—	0.7 ± 1.2	0.2 ± 0.9	1.1 ± 0.4	—
		Flexion–extension under axial load (supine)	—	—	0.7 ± 1.2	0.5 ± 0.5	0.9 ± 0.5	—
Mousavian et al. (2019)[30]	10	Flexion–extension	—	—	—	0.70 [1.6–−0.10]	—	—
Wong et al. (2021)[31]	58	Flexion–extension	—	—	−1.2 ± 0.6	0.1 ± 0.6	—	—

(continued on next page)

Table 1
(*continued*)

Study	n	Task	Rotational Range of Motion (Degrees)			Translational Range of Motion (mm)		
			Sagittal Plane (Dorsiflexion–Plantarflexion)	Coronal Plane (Eversion–Inversion)	Transverse Plane (External/Internal Rotation)	Sagittal Plane (Anterior–Posterior)	Coronal Plane (Medial–Lateral)	Transverse Plane (Superior–Inferior)
Bi-Plane Fluoroscopy								
Wang et al. (2015)[32]	16	Walking (stance phase)	2.98 ± 1.10	5.94 ± 1.52	5.99 ± 2.0	3.86 ± 1.65	2.63 ± 1.05	4.12 ± 1.53
Pitcairn et al. (2020)[33]	2	Walking	4.0 ± 1.7	9.0 ± 2.2	3.4 ± 1.0	—	—	—
		Running	2.9 ± 1.1	6.6 ± 1.4	3.0 ± 1.25	—	—	—
		Side-to-side single leg push off	3.4 ± 1.6	8.1 ± 0.7	2.3 ± 1.1	—	—	—
		Front-to-back single leg push off	2.9 ± 0.5	7.8 ± 3.3	4.0 ± 2.4	—	—	—
		Vertical jump	3.0 ± 0.4	14.3 ± 4.4	3.0 ± 1.0	—	—	—
		Forward single leg hop	2.8 ± 0.7	9.4 ± 1.9	2.8 ± 0.6	—	—	—
		Lateral single leg hop	3.0 ± 0.4	10.8 ± 3.8	2.7 ± 0.5	—	—	—
Hogg-Cornejo et al. (2020)[34]	6	Calf raise	1.3 ± 0.3	1.7 ± 1.0	8.1 ± 3.3	2.8 ± 1.4	1.7 ± 0.9	1.9 ± 0.8
		Squat	0.8 ± 0.2	1.0 ± 0.2	4.7 ± 2.8	2.2 ± 1.2	1.2 ± 0.6	2.1 ± 0.8
		Torso twist	1.4 ± 0.9	1.7 ± 1.0	8.8 ± 2.5	3.3 ± 2.2	1.5 ± 0.5	2.1 ± 0.7
		Box jump	1.7 ± 0.7	1.4 ± 0.5	9.4 ± 3.5	3.2 ± 1.0	1.7 ± 1.0	2.5 ± 0.9

[a] Dashes indicate that the study did not report data for that direction of motion. All values are mean and standard deviation, except for bracketed values that represent 95% confidence intervals.
[b] Results include direction with plantarflexion, inversion, and internal rotation being positive.
[c] Range of motion extrapolated from reported results.

both joint posture and bone position. The lack of standard reference frame for reporting ankle motion also makes comparisons across studies difficult.[37]

However, the variability in reported fibular motion may point to clinically relevant, subject-specific differences. Subject-specific differences in fibular motion were proposed by Barnett and Napier,[12] who described three classes of fibulae based on proximal tibiofibular joint morphology. More recently, in an *in vivo* study of 40 young adults, Okazaki and colleagues[36] found that changes in tibiofibular syndesmosis width during activity vary with sex and body mass. Owing to changes in laxity, syndesmosis width also significantly varies throughout the menstrual cycle.[38] These studies suggest individual fibula motion depends on a variety of factors. How to effectively consider subject-specific factors when evaluating fibula function and dysfunction remains an open clinical question.

Healthy Ankle Contact Mechanics

The historically quoted rule of thumb is that the fibula bears one-sixth (i.e., 16.7%) of the static load transmitted acros the ankle during weight-bearing.[39] However, other cadaveric studies suggest this is an overestimation, as they report that on average the fibula bears only 6% to 12% of the load, and the magnitude varies with ankle posture.[40–44] The fact that fibula loading varies with posture hints at the complexity of loading experienced in the ankle syndesmosis.

Within the ankle syndesmosis, forces are transmitted through articular joint surfaces and soft tissue constraints (**Fig. 2**). The complexity with which forces are distributed across the tibiotalar, tibiofibular, and talofibular articulations is matched by the complexity of the involved articular surface geometry. In addition, muscle, ligament, and articular forces all change dynamically during activity. Activating a muscle or stretching a ligament will alter the distribution of forces throughout the ankle joint complex.

A large number of cadaveric studies have examined contact mechanics in the healthy ankle by measuring contact area and/or contact pressure. These studies generally assume that decreased contact area is associated with increased pressure

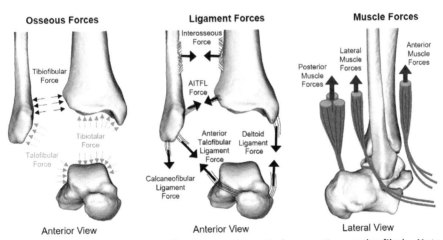

Fig. 2. Illustration of the osseous, ligament, and muscle forces acting on the fibula. Note, muscle forces are depicted using a simplified representation of muscle compartments. Also, the torques that occur due to these three-dimensional forces acting at a distance from the joint axes of rotation are not shown.

(force per unit area); however, this assumption only holds under constant load. Thus, caution must be taken when interpreting these studies, as findings may not readily extrapolate to dynamic activities with varying loads (e.g., walking, running). In addition, most studies focus on the tibiotalar articulation, or more specifically the talar dome (see Leardini and colleagues[45] and Brockett and Chapman[46] for review). Here, to understand loading across the healthy syndesmosis, we focus on studies that include talofibular articulation. To the best of our knowledge, contact mechanics at the tibiofibular joint have not been measured.

Calhoun and colleagues[47] performed one of the first cadaveric studies that measured contact area and pressure on all three facets of the talus during simulated walking postures in cadavers. On the basis of data from five specimens, they concluded the loads across the talocrural joint during walking are distributed such that the talar dome bears 77% to 90% of the total load, whereas the medial and lateral facets, respectively, bear 9% to 22% and 0.5% to 10.5%.[47] The medial facet experienced the largest loads during combined dorsiflexion and inversion, whereas the lateral facet experienced the largest loads during combined dorsiflexion and eversion. As the healthy ankle moved from platarflexion to dorsiflexion, the contact area on the talar dome increased. These findings indicate that dorsiflexion has greater joint congruity and stability than other ankle postures.[47] The qualitative description provided by Calhoun and colleagues[47] is generally corroborated by Kura and colleagues[48] and Michelson and colleagues.[49] However, quantitative comparison across studies is challenging due to differences in applied loads, postures, and measurement techniques.

In contrast, based on data from 10 specimens, Millington and colleagues[50] report opposite findings for talofibular contact, stating that talofibular contact area is larger in supination (inversion) than pronation (eversion). Note, we are reporting this result using the terminology adopted by Millington and colleagues,[50] although they state their definition of pronation/supination matches the definition of eversion/inversion reported by Calhoun and colleagues.[47] The small contact area in pronation is explained by a small localized contact between the distal fibula tip and lateral talar facet in this posture. Millington and colleagues[50] used a stereophotographic technique, which unlike pressure-sensitive films and force transducers, enables precise measurement across curved surfaces with complex 3D topography. Differences in measurement techniques may account for the reported differences in contact mechanics.

Summary

Overall, research indicates that the fibula experiences complex six degree-of-freedom motion. Although small, the magnitude and direction of the rotations and translations vary with task. Consequently, loading patterns also vary with task. In healthy ankles, the tibiofibular articulation between the distal fibula and lateral facet of the talus primarily experiences loading during inversion and eversion. To what extent these loading patterns and the motions associated with them are subject-specific is open to debate. But, ankle mechanics are highly dependent upon the morphology of the tibia, fibula, and talus.

SYNDESMOSIS INJURY
Clinical Presentation of Syndesmosis Injury

Syndesmosis injuries may occur in isolation or in combination with bone fractures and ankle lateral ligament sprains. The mechanism of injury classically involves an external rotation of the talus within the ankle mortise, most commonly occurring when the foot was planted in ankle dorsiflexion. During this archetypal injury mechanism, the talus leverages against the fibula causing external rotation, posterior and lateral displacement, and distal translation.

The severity of syndesmosis ligamentous injury ranges from low-grade isolated sprain of the AITFL to catastrophic rupture of all syndesmosis ligaments with frank displacement of the fibula away from the tibia. Medial ankle deltoid ligament injury often accompanies severe syndesmosis injuries. Nonstressed radiographs and stress maneuvers are used to assess instability and grade injury severity.

In general, there is consistent correspondence between an anatomic point of tenderness and injury to the named structure in that location when viewed on magnetic resonance or ultrasound imaging or when viewed by ankle arthroscopy. Likewise, the severity of injury corresponds to the duration of recovery.

Ankle fractures may produce a mixed pattern of syndesmosis ligament sprain and bone injury. Fracture patterns include ligament avulsions of one or more tubercles, malleolar fractures, and ankle joint displacement, which also occurs along a spectrum from anatomically aligned to frank dislocation.

Syndesmosis Injury Disrupts Fibular Motion

When a ligament is injured its function is compromised, thereby affecting the motion of the bones to which it connects. Although this is intuitively understood, quantifying how ligament injury alters bone motion is challenging, particularly in the case of injuries involving multiple ligaments, such as those involving the ankle syndesmosis. In an effort to understand how high ankle sprains influence fibular motion, a variety of cadaveric studies have simulated syndesmosis injury via ligament sectioning. This research was evaluated by two recent systematic reviews.[51,52] Note, these reviews have similar aims and the same publication year (2021), but only two studies are included in both.

Spennacchio and colleagues[52] reviewed 14 studies to identify sequential ligament injuries that result in syndesmosis instability. The findings indicate an isolated rupture of either the AITFL or deltoid ligament compromises the dynamic stability of the syndesmosis. Given that most of the measured changes in fibular motion were provoked by external rotation, the authors conclude external rotation stress testing is an important diagnostic tool.[52]

Khambete and colleagues[51] reviewed 12 studies to understand how individual syndesmosis ligaments contribute to stability, particularly in response to external rotation forces. The findings indicate that the interosseous membrane may be the strongest and stiffest of the syndesmosis ligaments; however, the AITFL and PITFL are critical for resisting external and internal rotation forces, respectively. Based on their findings, the authors postulate the location of fixation constructs should be chosen along ligament planes based on the direction of stability to be restored. Biomechanical studies supporting this hypothesis are still needed.[51]

Taken together, these reviews highlight that the evidence regarding how syndesmosis injury impacts fibular kinematics is dominated by cadaveric studies. Across these studies, the mechanical explanations for observed kinematic changes lack unity. This is partially explained by sectioning differences. For example, when using an anterior-to-posterior cutting order, the PITFL was found to control fibular translation, but when using a posterior-to-anterior cutting order, the AITFL was found to control fibular translation.[53] Cadaveric studies also cannot fully capture the spectrum of ligament injury. Ultimately, in vivo studies are needed to elucidate changes in fibular kinematics associated with syndesmotic injury and understand how those kinematics should be considered during diagnosis and treatment.

Syndesmosis Injury Alters Ankle Contact Mechanics

Syndesmosis injury alters the arthrokinematics of the fibula, thereby altering how forces are transmitted across the talocrural joint. This relationship between arthrokinematics and force is well illustrated by the classic work of Ramsey and Hamilton.[54] In this work, injuries that result in mortise widening were studied by measuring changes in contact area with lateral displacement of the talus; the first 1 mm of lateral displacement corresponded to a 42% decrease in contact area, with each subsequent displacement reducing contact area by increasingly smaller amounts.[54] This result has been affirmed by several studies[55–58] and highlights the importance of maintaining the anatomic integrity of the ankle mortise to maintain healthy joint loading.

Given that mortise widening is not necessarily representative of all syndesmosis injuries, studies have evaluated joint contact and ligament mechanics in the presence of simulated high ankle sprains. For example, Burns and colleagues[59] sequentially simulated healthy, AITFL rupture, syndesmosis injury without deltoid rupture (AITFL, PITFL, and interosseous ligaments sectioned), and complete syndesmosis rupture (AITFL, PITFL, interosseous, and deltoid ligaments sectioned) in 10 specimens. Their results highlight the critical importance of the deltoid ligament, as syndesmosis injury without deltoid rupture was associated with an average tibiofibular widening of only 0.24 mm and there was not an associated increase in tibiotalar contact area or peak pressure.[59] In contrast, complete syndesmosis injury with deltoid rupture was associated with 0.73 mm of tibiofibular widening, 39% decrease in contact area, and a 42% increase in peak pressure. Thus, syndesmotic diastasis of less than 1 mm can negatively impact ankle joint dynamics.[59] This lends credence to the clinical belief that even small magnitudes of fibula malreduction can be problematic.

In a similar study, Hunt and colleagues[60] evaluated syndesmosis injury via sequential ligament sectioning and measured contact area and pressure in eight specimens. Measurements were recorded under both axial load and axial load in combination with an external rotation torque.[60] Their results confirm that syndesmosis injury alters contact mechanics and that the deltoid ligament is important for stability, whereas the analysis of external rotation importantly expands prior work. Specifically, Hunt and colleagues[60] found that external rotation significantly displaced the fibula and talus, which subsequently caused a shift in the center of pressure and decrease in the contact area. This illustrates the importance of limiting external rotation during rehabilitation to allow ligament healing while minimizing abnormal joint loading.[60]

Given that fibula fractures commonly occur in conjunction with syndesmosis injuries, the substantial literature on fibula fracture contact mechanics warrants a brief summary. Cadaveric studies (e.g.,[57,61–63]) indicate that fibula shortening, fibula malrotation, and/or fibula displacement negatively impacts talocrural contact mechanics. Yet, an *in vivo* clinical study that indirectly assessed ankle joint loading by measuring subchondral bone mineralization in the tali of 72 fracture patients concluded that fracture gaps up to 3 mm do not alter talocrural joint load.[64] Given that this study excluded patients with evident talar shift of 1 mm or more, the results suggest that maintaining talar position may be one of the most important factors to consider when treating syndesmosis injuries.

Summary

Overall, the research suggests that syndesmosis injury alters both motion and loading across the talocrural joint. Although many postulates that these altered mechanics contribute to the development of osteochondral lesions and osteoarthritis,[60] this relationship has not been explicitly shown. Given osteoarthritis is a complex disease that affects the joint as an organ system, alterations in joint mechanics are likely only one of many contributing factors. Therefore, the goal of treatment of syndesmosis injuries is restoration of anatomic alignment and healthy joint mechanics.

REPAIRED SYNDESMOSIS
Clinical Management of Syndesmosis Injuries

In broad terms, syndesmosis injuries with a stable syndesmotic joint are treated nonsurgically. The acute pain, swelling, and inflammation are managed with rest, ice, elevation, compression, and protected weight-bearing, most commonly in a boot or cast (see Williams and colleagues[65] for review). Physical therapy is initiated as soon as permitted by the absence of renewed pain or swelling when performing exercises. The rehabilitation process advances as the patient tolerates until achieving a return to usual activities or sports participation. In elite athletes, there is a lower threshold for surgical intervention to expedite recovery.

Surgical treatment is indicated to anatomically restore joint alignment, inclusive of repairing displaced fractures, and stabilization of the syndesmotic joint. Ankle syndesmosis surgery takes on many forms including arthroscopy, anatomic ligament repair, fracture repair, and fixation across the ankle syndesmosis. Of relevance to the biomechanics discussion below, syndesmosis fixation is classically performed using rigid 3.5 or 4.5 mm screws inserted from the fibula side.[4] Although no longer the predominant surgical method due to advances in flexible fixation and soft tissue repair/reconstructive methods, such rigid fixation is necessary when the fibula is fractured higher up the leg in a length-unstable spiral or multi-fragmented pattern. Compared with rigid syndesmosis fixation, flexible fixation is commonly achieved using a high-tensile strength suture tunneled through the fibula and tibia that is tensioned between metallic buttons on the outsides of each bone. This fixation construct, or suture-button, reduces the incidence of later implant removal for pain, implant failure, or implant migration compared with screw fixation. Regardless of fixation construct, postoperative management of the syndesmosis largely parallels the process for nonsurgical treatment but with a longer time course.

Restoring Native Kinematics Remains a Treatment Challenge

Studies evaluating how nonoperative treatment affects fibula motion are limited.[66,67] Lamer and colleagues[66] showed in a cadaveric model of syndesmosis injury that a controlled ankle motion (CAM) walking boot actually increased fibular external rotation when an axial load was applied. This is concerning, as excess fibular rotation in a vulnerable ankle could lead to poor healing and ongoing pain from repetitive strain on the healing ligament. Further work examining high-ankle sprain taping in a cadaver model found no difference in tibiofibular kinematics between specimens with or without tape.[67] These studies highlight a need for *in vivo* work characterizing the mechanical effects of conservative treatment.

Intuitively, surgically repairing the syndesmosis by rigidly fixing the fibula to the tibia alters tibiofibular motion. Both *in vivo* and cadaveric studies have confirmed this (e.g.,[53,68–79]). For example, in a small prospective study of five adults treated with a syndesmotic screw, AITFL reconstruction, and subsequent screw removal, Beumer and colleagues[68] report postoperative restrictions in fibular motion. Specifically, when comparing fibular motion during an external rotation stress test between patients 3-month postoperative and asymptomatic controls, medial translation, posterior translation, and external rotation were significantly smaller, whereas cranial translation was significantly larger.[68] However, the change in motion is small. Differences between average preoperative and postoperative measurements of fibular translation and rotation may be less than 1 mm and 1.5°.[68]

Flexible fixation obviously allows more fibular motion than rigid fixation, but it may also result in more motion than the intact ankle. Cadaveric studies indicate that when compared with intact ankles, syndesmosis fixation with a single suture-button is associated with higher anterior–posterior translation,[69,71–73] internal rotation,[53] and external rotation.[70,73] Although there is little consensus regarding the direction of change, studies consistently note a significant increase in fibular motion. Similarly, syndesmosis fixation with a double suture-button does not result in fibular translations that match the intact ankle.[53] Given that these studies were performed in cadaver specimens, it is impossible to know whether these findings show desirable mimicry of fibular motion or merely suggest that some degree of instability persists before healing.

To be clear, neither rigid nor flexible fixation restores intact ankle kinematics. Studies suggest that screws better restore physiologic fibular translations, whereas suture-buttons better restore physiologic fibular rotations.[78,79] But, a critical evaluation of the evidence does not result in a clear consensus regarding the best fixation construct.

Although the best fixation construct remains uncertain, anatomic repair of the ligaments can be important. Cadaveric studies indicate that reconstruction or repair of the AITFL enhances stability of the syndesmosis (e.g.,[70,80–82]). For example, in a recent study of 12 cadaveric specimens, Jamieson and colleagues[70] showed that repair of the AITFL with or without suture-tape augmentation resulted in fibular motion that was not statistically different than the intact ankle. However, talar motion was significantly different than the intact state.[70] Other studies (e.g.,[81]) corroborate this finding: soft tissue repair may restore fibular, but not talar motion.

Treatment Does Not Fully Restore Healthy Ankle Contact Mechanics

Syndesmosis fixation increases tibiotalar joint force relative to the injured state,[73,83] but this increase does not necessarily restore the tibiotalar joint force of a healthy joint.[73,83,84] For example, both LaMothe and colleagues [73] and Kelly and colleagues[83] report a decrease in tibiotalar joint force following syndesmosis fixation compared with an intact ankle. Goetz and colleagues[84] confirm that this decrease in force on the talar dome results in an increase in force on the medial and lateral facets of the talus; however, this increase only reaches statistical significance for some ankle postures (neutral and dorsiflexion). It should be noted that the experimental design of these studies varied, with key differences in injury model and fixation construct.

Given the widespread debate between rigid versus flexible fixation, multiple studies have examined how the choice of implant influences ankle joint loading.[73,77,85] LaMothe and colleagues [73] conclude that screw fixation without a clamp is superior to both screw fixation with a clamp and suture-button fixation, although all three fixation techniques negatively impact tibiotalar joint mechanics. In contrast, Pang and colleagues[77] conclude that two 3.5 mm screws or two suture-buttons are both adequate due to similarities in the imposed tibiotalar joint mechanics, whereas Graff and colleagues[85] conclude that use of one screw provides stronger fixation than one suture-button because it imposes both a larger force and larger contact area across the tibiofibular joint. Again, clear conclusions across studies are challenging due to differences in experimental design.

In the context of rigid syndesmosis fixation, studies have examined how differences in number of screws (1 vs 2 screws)[83,84] screw size (3.5 vs 4.5 mm),[86] and number of engaged cortices (tricortical vs quadricortical)[86] influence ankle joint loading. Tibiotalar and tibiofibular contact mechanics were similar with one versus two screws,[83,84] suggesting that the number of screws selected for fixation should be guided by considerations other than restoring joint contact mechanics. Similarly, although 4.5 mm screws are technically more resistant to shear compared with 3.5 mm screws,[87] neither screw size nor the number of engaged cortices significantly alters forces on the distal fibula.[86] It is important to note that these studies focus on measuring contact forces at the articular surface, not forces within the fibula and tibia near the implanted screws. Thus, in combination with work examining screw failure modes, these studies suggest that avoiding high forces on the screw and therefore avoiding screw failure should guide screw selection, instead of consideration of distal fibula contact forces.

A few studies have also examined to what extent simulated malreduction influences tibiotalar contact mechanics.[83,88] Notably, in a study of six specimens, Pereira and colleagues[88] evaluated the effects of mortise widening in the presence of rigid screw fixation. They conclude screw fixation initially changes tibiotalar contact mechanics, but mortise widening up to 4 mm does not further change those mechanics in screw fixated cadaveric specimens without simulated deltoid ligament rupture.[88] Similarly, in a study of eight specimens, Kelly and colleagues[83] conclude that anterior malreduction, simulated as 5-mm anterior displacement of the fibula, results in similar contact mechanics as anatomic reduction. Given the small sample sizes, neither is sufficiently powered to claim there is no difference between anatomic reduction and malreduction. In addition, these studies seem to contradict kinematic studies demonstrating that malreduction significantly affects fibular motion,[89] as a change in motion is likely to result in a change in joint loading. Regardless, currently available evidence suggests that the negative effect of fixation itself on contact mechanics may be larger than that of malreduction.

Summary

Overall, syndesmosis fixation changes motion and load across the tibiotalar, tibiofibular, and talofibular joints. However, given the complexity of syndesmosis injury patterns and the absence of a universally accepted fixation construct, clear conclusions regarding the magnitude of these changes are muddled by differences in simulated injury, simulated surgical fixation, and experimental design. In addition, although a limited number of studies have examined fibula motion following syndesmosis fixation, all studies of surgically-induced syndesmosis contact mechanics rely on cadaveric data. Thus, to what extent detrimental changes in contact mechanics exist *in vivo* remains unknown. To the best of our knowledge, there are only two studies to examine plantar pressure distribution during gait following syndesmosis repair. Both indicate that loading changes postoperatively.[90,91] To what extent these postoperative changes in gait are protective versus detrimental to internal joint loading is an open question that warrants investigation.

THE ROLE OF COMPUTATIONAL MODELS: A BRIEF COMMENTARY

In a manner similar to cadaveric experiments, computational models have been used to investigate healthy ankle mechanics, the impact of syndesmosis injury, and the effect of surgical fixation (e.g.,[92–105]). The primary advantage of computational modeling studies is the ability to precisely control variables. This allows direct comparison of study conditions (e.g., number of screws, screw size) in the absence of confounding variables (e.g., morphologic differences across specimens, inadvertent malreduction due to screw placement). However, computational models are limited by small sample size, as most finite element models are based on the anatomy of a single individual, and lack of validation, as few computational modeling studies of the ankle syndesmosis include explicit experimental validation (see Liacouras and Wayne[95] for an example of a syndesmosis study with experimental validation).

To provide an example, in one of the most comprehensive finite element modeling studies of the ankle syndesmosis to date, Alastuey-Lopez and colleagues[92] provide quantitative data comparing 23 fixation constructs to the intact and injured syndesmosis (25 total finite element models). The fixation constructs vary in number of screws (one vs two 3.5 mm screws), engaged cortices (tricorticol vs quadcorticol fixation), inter-screw distance (10, 15, and 18 mm), suture-button configuration (one vs two parallel vs two divergent), and suture-button pretension (20, 30, 40, 80, and 100N). The design of this study illustrates the potential power of computational models for systematically studying many clinically important variables. However, the conclusions that can be drawn from this study are limited by the fact that the authors report only two metrics, syndesmosis widening and maximum stress on the fixation construct, and provide no validation beyond qualitative comparison to prior cadaveric studies. Thus, even though multiple fixation constructs (namely one single tricorticol screw, double quadricorticol screws with 18 mm inter-screw distance, and most single and double suture-button configurations) resulted in a similar syndesmosis width to the intact ankle, it is unknown from this study alone to what extent these configurations do or do not influence joint contact mechanics or clinical outcomes.

Other computational studies have directly evaluated joint contact mechanics following syndesmosis injury and repair (e.g.,[93–96,102]). These studies expand the conclusions of cadaveric studies in two important ways. First, injury and repair alter contact mechanics between not only the talus, tibia, and fibula, but also the talus, calcaneus, and navicular.[94–96] Second, the presence of synovial fluid decreases the magnitude and changes the distribution of stress on the talocrural joint.[93] Simultaneously measuring talocrural, subtalar, and talonavicular contact mechanics and/or incorporating the effects of synovial fluid into a cadaveric model is exceedingly difficult. Thus, high-quality computational models have the potential to play an important role in expanding our knowledge of the ankle syndesmosis.

DISCUSSION

Regardless of whether the ankle syndesmosis is intact, injured, or repaired, the fibula moves in complex ways. The magnitude of rotation and translation is small. But, even small changes in the position or movement of the fibula will alter how forces propagate through the adjacent joints of the ankle and foot.

Altered fibular mechanics likely impact patient outcomes. This conclusion is suggested by an early in vivo case series by Scranton and colleagues,[106] which found that restriction of fibula motion is associated with ankle pain when weight-bearing. However, the restriction was caused by tibiofibular synostosis, which is not necessarily equivalent to syndesmotic fixation. In the context of syndesmosis fixation, there is a paucity of in vivo data examining fibular mechanics in syndesmosis patients. But, measurements of fibular motion do indicate kinematics are highly variable across individuals and often include at least some outliers. Thus, it is reasonable to postulate that altered mechanics contribute to poor outcomes for at least some patients. However, to understand the relationship between fibula mechanics and outcomes, *in vivo* data evaluating mechanics and outcomes in a single, patient cohort is needed.

Future work should also aim to expand our understanding of the patient-specific nature of fibular mechanics. Given that the diameter, curvature, and anatomic position of the fibula are not bilaterally symmetric within individuals,[8,9] there are likely patient-specific and potentially even limb-specific differences in fibular mechanics of clinical relevance. In addition, muscle strength and structure are known to vary across individuals, but little is known about the effects of muscles on the fibula. Both *in vivo* and computational modeling studies are primed to fill this gap in knowledge and inform innovations related to patient-specific syndesmosis clinical care.

SUMMARY

- Syndesmosis injuries are complex, often involving multiple ligaments and concomitant injuries.
- Subject-specific factors, such as bone morphology, injury pattern, injury severity, and fixation approach, impact fibula mechanics.
- An ideal fixation construct and/or surgical technique capable of matching fibula mechanics between intact and repaired syndesmoses has not yet been identified.
- Arthrokinematics and loading patterns across the foot and ankle change in the presence of syndesmosis injury and after repair. However, the clinical consequences of these changes are unknown.
- There is a need for *in vivo* studies examining the relationship between syndesmosis biomechanics and patient-reported outcomes.

CLINICS CARE POINTS

- When treating the ankle syndesmosis, native fibular mechanics should be restored to the largest extent possible, as altered fibular mechanics may negatively impact patient outcomes.

- Biomechanical considerations alone are insufficient to identify the best surgical approach for treating the ankle syndesmosis, as there is a lack of consensus regarding how different fixation approaches affect fibular mechanics.

- Because both injury and surgical fixation may result in residual syndesmosis pathomechanics due to altered fibula position and/or motion, these factors should be evaluated in the patient with persisting pain or functional impairment after treatment.

- A patient-specific treatment approach is advised to account for differences in morphology, injury severity, and functional goals.

REFERENCES

1. Barnett CH, Napier JR. The form and mobility of the fibula in metatherian mammals. J Anat 1953;87(2):207–13.
2. Heifner JJ, Kilgore JE, Nichols JA, et al. Syndesmosis Injury Contributes a Large Negative Effect on Clinical Outcomes: A Systematic Review. Foot Ankle Spec 2022. https://doi.org/10.1177/19386400211067865. 19386400211067864.
3. Hermans JJ, Beumer A, de Jong TAW, et al. Anatomy of the distal tibiofibular syndesmosis in adults: a pictorial essay with a multimodality approach. J Anat 2010;217(6):633–45. https://doi.org/10.1111/j.1469-7580.2010.01302.x.

4. Zalavras C, Thordarson D. Ankle syndesmotic injury. J Am Acad Orthop Surg 2007;15(6):330–9. https://doi.org/10.5435/00124635-200706000-00002.

5. Boszczyk A, Kwapisz S, Krümmel M, et al. Correlation of Incisura Anatomy With Syndesmotic Malreduction. Foot Ankle Int 2018;39(3):369–75. https://doi.org/10.1177/1071100717744332.

6. Croft S, Furey A, Stone C, et al. Radiographic evaluation of the ankle syndesmosis. Can J Surg 2015;58(1):58–62. https://doi.org/10.1503/cjs.004214.

7. Souleiman F, Heilemann M, Hennings R, et al. A standardized approach for exact CT-based three-dimensional position analysis in the distal tibiofibular joint. BMC Med Imaging 2021;21(1):41. https://doi.org/10.1186/s12880-021-00570-y.

8. Kubik JF, Rollick NC, Bear J, et al. Assessment of malreduction standards for the syndesmosis in bilateral CT scans of uninjured ankles. Bone Joint J 2021;103-B(1):178–83. https://doi.org/10.1302/0301-620X.103B1.BJJ-2020-0844.R1.

9. Tümer N, Arbabi V, Gielis WP, et al. Three-dimensional analysis of shape variations and symmetry of the fibula, tibia, calcaneus and talus. J Anat 2019;234(1):132–44. https://doi.org/10.1111/joa.12900.

10. Weinert CR, McMaster JH, Ferguson RJ. Dynamic function of the human fibula. Am J Anat 1973;138(2):145–9. https://doi.org/10.1002/aja.1001380202.

11. ASHHURST APC, BROMER RS. Classification and mechanism of fractures of the leg bones involving the ankle: based on a study of three hundred cases from the episcopal hospital. Arch Surg 1922;4(1):51–129. https://doi.org/10.1001/archsurg.1922.01110100060003.

12. Barnett CH, Napier JR. The axis of rotation at the ankle joint in man; its influence upon the form of the talus and the mobility of the fibula. J Anat 1952;86(1):1–9.

13. Bolin H. The fibula and its relationship the tibia and talus in injuries of the ankle due to forced external rotation. Acta Radiol 1961;56:439–48. https://doi.org/10.3109/00016926109172839.

14. Lundberg A. Kinematics of the ankle and foot. In vivo roentgen stereophotogrammetry. Acta Orthop Scand Suppl 1989;233:1–24. https://doi.org/10.1186/1757-1146-5-s1-k5.

15. Svensson OK, Lundberg A, Walheirn G, et al. In vivo fibular motions during various movements of the ankle. Clin Biomech (Bristol, Avon) 1989;4(3):155–60. https://doi.org/10.1016/0268-0033(89)90019-3.

16. Close JR. Some applications of the functional anatomy of the ankle joint. J Bone Joint Surg Am 1956;38-A(4):761–81.

17. Leardini A, O'Connor JJ, Catani F, et al. Kinematics of the human ankle complex in passive flexion; a single degree of freedom system. J Biomech 1999;32(2):111–8. https://doi.org/10.1016/s0021-9290(98)00157-2.

18. Soavi R, Girolami M, Loreti I, et al. The mobility of the proximal tibio-fibular joint. A Roentgen Stereophotogrammetric Analysis on six cadaver specimens. Foot Ankle Int 2000;21(4):336–42. https://doi.org/10.1177/107110070002100411.

19. Bozkurt M, Tonuk E, Elhan A, et al. Axial rotation and mediolateral translation of the fibula during passive plantarflexion. Foot Ankle Int 2008;29(5):502–7. https://doi.org/10.3113/FAI-2008-0502.

20. Hu WK, Chen DW, Li B, et al. Motion of the distal tibiofibular syndesmosis under different loading patterns: A biomechanical study. J Orthop Surg (Hong Kong) 2019;27(2). https://doi.org/10.1177/2309499019842879. 2309499019842879.

21. Kärrholm J, Hansson LI, Selvik G. Mobility of the lateral malleolus. A roentgen stereophotogrammetric analysis. Acta Orthop Scand 1985;56(6):479–83. https://doi.org/10.3109/17453678508993039.

22. Ahl T, Dalén N, Lundberg A, et al. Mobility of the ankle mortise. A roentgen ster-eophotogrammetric analysis. Acta Orthop Scand 1987;58(4):401–2. https://doi.org/10.3109/17453678709146365.
23. Beumer A, Valstar ER, Garling EH, et al. Kinematics of the distal tibiofibular syn-desmosis: radiostereometry in 11 normal ankles. Acta Orthop Scand 2003; 74(3):337–43. https://doi.org/10.1080/00016470310014283.
24. Arndt A, Wolf P, Liu A, et al. Intrinsic foot kinematics measured in vivo during the stance phase of slow running. J Biomech 2007;40(12):2672–8. https://doi.org/10.1016/j.jbiomech.2006.12.009.
25. Lundgren P, Nester C, Liu A, et al. Invasive in vivo measurement of rear-, mid-and forefoot motion during walking. Gait Posture 2008;28(1):93–100. https://doi.org/10.1016/j.gaitpost.2007.10.009.
26. Lepojärvi S, Niinimäki J, Pakarinen H, et al. Rotational Dynamics of the Normal Distal Tibiofibular Joint With Weight-Bearing Computed Tomography. Foot Ankle Int 2016;37(6):627–35. https://doi.org/10.1177/1071100716634757.
27. Hoogervorst P, Working ZM, El Naga AN, et al. In Vivo CT Analysis of Physiolog-ical Fibular Motion at the Level of the Ankle Syndesmosis During Plantigrade Weightbearing. Foot Ankle Spec 2019;12(3):233–7. https://doi.org/10.1177/1938640018782602.
28. Malhotra K, Welck M, Cullen N, et al. The effects of weight bearing on the distal tibiofibular syndesmosis: A study comparing weight bearing-CT with conven-tional CT. Foot Ankle Surg 2019;25(4):511–6. https://doi.org/10.1016/j.fas.2018.03.006.
29. Jend HH, Ney R, Heller M. Evaluation of tibiofibular motion under load condi-tions by computed tomography. J Orthop Res 1985;3(4):418–23. https://doi.org/10.1002/jor.1100030404.
30. Mousavian A, Shakoor D, Hafezi-Nejad N, et al. Tibiofibular syndesmosis in asymptomatic ankles: initial kinematic analysis using four-dimensional CT. Clin Radiol 2019;74(7):571.e1–8. https://doi.org/10.1016/j.crad.2019.03.015, e8.
31. Wong MT, Wiens C, Lamothe J, et al. Four-Dimensional CT Analysis of Normal Syndesmotic Motion. Foot Ankle Int 2021;42(11):1491–501. https://doi.org/10.1177/10711007211015204.
32. Wang C, Yang J, Wang S, et al. Three-dimensional motions of distal syndesmo-sis during walking. J Orthop Surg Res 2015;10:166. https://doi.org/10.1186/s13018-015-0306-5.
33. Pitcairn S, Kromka J, Hogan M, et al. Validation and application of dynamic biplane radiography to study in vivo ankle joint kinematics during high-demand activities. J Biomech 2020;103:109696. https://doi.org/10.1016/j.jbiomech.2020.109696.
34. Hogg-Cornejo V, Hunt KJ, Bartolomei J, et al. Normal Kinematics of the Syndes-mosis and Ankle Mortise During Dynamic Movements. Foot Ankle Orthop 2020; 5(3). https://doi.org/10.1177/2473011420933007. 2473011420933007.
35. Alves-da-Silva T, Guerra-Pinto F, Matias R, et al. Kinematics of the proximal tibio-fibular joint is influenced by ligament integrity, knee and ankle mobility: an exploratory cadaver study. Knee Surg Sports Traumatol Arthrosc 2019;27(2): 405–11. https://doi.org/10.1007/s00167-018-5070-8.
36. Okazaki M, Kaneko M, Ishida Y, et al. Gender difference in distance of tibiofib-ular syndesmosis to joint dynamics of lower extremities during squat. J Physiol Sci 2015;65(2):165–70. https://doi.org/10.1007/s12576-015-0355-x.
37. Lenz AL, Strobel MA, Anderson AM, et al. Assignment of local coordinate sys-tems and methods to calculate tibiotalar and subtalar kinematics: A systematic

review. J Biomech 2021;120:110344. https://doi.org/10.1016/j.jbiomech.2021.110344.

38. Okazaki M, Kaneko M, Ishida Y, et al. Changes in the Width of the Tibiofibular Syndesmosis Related to Lower Extremity Joint Dynamics and Neuromuscular Coordination on Drop Landing During the Menstrual Cycle. Orthop J Sports Med 2017; 5(9). https://doi.org/10.1177/2325967117724753. 2325967117724753.

39. Lambert KL. The weight-bearing function of the fibula. A strain gauge study. J Bone Joint Surg Am 1971;53(3):507–13.

40. Goh JC, Mech AM, Lee EH, et al. Biomechanical study on the load-bearing characteristics of the fibula and the effects of fibular resection. Clin Orthop Relat Res 1992;279:223–8.

41. Funk JR, Rudd RW, Kerrigan JR, et al. The effect of tibial curvature and fibular loading on the tibia index. Traffic Inj Prev 2004;5(2):164–72. https://doi.org/10.1080/15389580490436069.

42. Wang Q, Whittle M, Cunningham J, et al. Fibula and its ligaments in load transmission and ankle joint stability. Clin Orthop Relat Res 1996;330:261–70. https://doi.org/10.1097/00003086-199609000-00034.

43. Takebe K, Nakagawa A, Minami H, et al. Role of the fibula in weight-bearing. Clin Orthop Relat Res 1984;184:289–92.

44. Segal D, Pick RY, Klein HA, et al. The role of the lateral malleolus as a stabilizing factor of the ankle joint: preliminary report. Foot Ankle 1981;2(1):25–9. https://doi.org/10.1177/107110078100200104.

45. Leardini A, O'Connor JJ, Catani F, et al. The role of the passive structures in the mobility and stability of the human ankle joint: a literature review. Foot Ankle Int 2000;21(7):602–15. https://doi.org/10.1177/107110070002100715.

46. Brockett CL, Chapman GJ. Biomechanics of the ankle. Orthop Trauma 2016; 30(3):232–8. https://doi.org/10.1016/j.mporth.2016.04.015.

47. Calhoun JH, Li F, Ledbetter BR, et al. A comprehensive study of pressure distribution in the ankle joint with inversion and eversion. Foot Ankle Int 1994;15(3): 125–33. https://doi.org/10.1177/107110079401500307.

48. Kura H, Kitaoka HB, Luo ZP, et al. Measurement of surface contact area of the ankle joint. Clin Biomech (Bristol, Avon) 1998;13(4–5):365–70. https://doi.org/10.1016/s0268-0033(98)00011-4.

49. Michelson JD, Checcone M, Kuhn T, et al. Intra-articular load distribution in the human ankle joint during motion. Foot Ankle Int 2001;22(3):226–33. https://doi.org/10.1177/107110070102200310.

50. Millington S, Grabner M, Wozelka R, et al. A stereophotographic study of ankle joint contact area. J Orthop Res 2007;25(11):1465–73. https://doi.org/10.1002/jor.20425.

51. Khambete P, Harlow E, Ina J, et al. Biomechanics of the Distal Tibiofibular Syndesmosis: A Systematic Review of Cadaveric Studies. Foot Ankle Orthop 2021; 6(2). https://doi.org/10.1177/24730114211012701. 24730114211012700.

52. Spennacchio P, Seil R, Gathen M, et al. Diagnosing instability of ligamentous syndesmotic injuries: A biomechanical perspective. Clin Biomech (Bristol, Avon) 2021;84:105312. https://doi.org/10.1016/j.clinbiomech.2021.105312.

53. Clanton TO, Williams BT, Backus JD, et al. Biomechanical Analysis of the Individual Ligament Contributions to Syndesmotic Stability. Foot Ankle Int 2017; 38(1):66–75. https://doi.org/10.1177/1071100716666277.

54. Ramsey PL, Hamilton W. Changes in tibiotalar area of contact caused by lateral talar shift. J Bone Joint Surg Am 1976;58(3):356–7.

55. Kimizuka M, Kurosawa H, Fukubayashi T. Load-bearing pattern of the ankle joint. Contact area and pressure distribution. Arch Orthop Trauma Surg (1978) 1980;96(1):45–9. https://doi.org/10.1007/BF01246141.

56. Moody ML, Koeneman J, Hettinger E, et al. The effects of fibular and talar displacement on joint contact areas about the ankle. Orthop Rev 1992;21(6): 741–4.

57. Thordarson DB, Motamed S, Hedman T, et al. The effect of fibular malreduction on contact pressures in an ankle fracture malunion model. J Bone Joint Surg Am 1997;79(12):1809–15. https://doi.org/10.2106/00004623-199712000-00006.

58. Lloyd J, Elsayed S, Hariharan K, et al. Revisiting the concept of talar shift in ankle fractures. Foot Ankle Int 2006;27(10):793–6. https://doi.org/10.1177/107110070602701006.

59. Burns WC, Prakash K, Adelaar R, et al. Tibiotalar joint dynamics: indications for the syndesmotic screw–a cadaver study. Foot Ankle 1993;14(3):153–8. https://doi.org/10.1177/107110079301400308.

60. Hunt KJ, Goeb Y, Behn AW, et al. Ankle Joint Contact Loads and Displacement With Progressive Syndesmotic Injury. Foot Ankle Int 2015;36(9):1095–103. https://doi.org/10.1177/1071100715583456.

61. Curtis MJ, Michelson JD, Urquhart MW, et al. Tibiotalar contact and fibular malunion in ankle fractures. A cadaver study. Acta Orthop Scand 1992;63(3):326–9. https://doi.org/10.3109/17453679209154793.

62. Harris J, Fallat L. Effects of isolated Weber B fibular fractures on the tibiotalar contact area. J Foot Ankle Surg 2004;43(1):3–9. https://doi.org/10.1053/j.jfas.2003.11.008.

63. Stroh DA, DeFontes K, Paez A, et al. Distal fibular malrotation and lateral ankle contact characteristics. Foot Ankle Surg 2019;25(1):90–3. https://doi.org/10.1016/j.fas.2017.09.001.

64. Deml C, Eichinger M, van Leeuwen WF, et al. Does intra-articular load distribution change after lateral malleolar fractures? An in vivo study comparing operative and nonoperative treatment. Injury 2017;48(4):854–60. https://doi.org/10.1016/j.injury.2017.02.035.

65. Williams GN, Allen EJ. Rehabilitation of syndesmotic (high) ankle sprains. Sports Health 2010;2(6):460–70. https://doi.org/10.1177/1941738110384573.

66. Lamer S, Hébert-Davies J, Dubé V, et al. Effect of a Controlled Ankle Motion Walking Boot on Syndesmotic Instability During Weightbearing: A Cadaveric Study. Orthop J Sports Med 2019;7(8). https://doi.org/10.1177/2325967119864018. 2325967119864018.

67. Lamer S, Hébert-Davies J, Dubé V, et al. The Effect of "High-ankle Sprain" Taping on Ankle Syndesmosis Congruity: A Cadaveric Study. Open Sports Sci J 2020;13(1). https://doi.org/10.2174/1875399X02013010123.

68. Beumer A, Valstar ER, Garling EH, et al. Kinematics before and after reconstruction of the anterior syndesmosis of the ankle: A prospective radiostereometric and clinical study in 5 patients. Acta Orthop 2005;76(5):713–20. https://doi.org/10.1080/17453670510041817.

69. Klitzman R, Zhao H, Zhang LQ, et al. Suture-button versus screw fixation of the syndesmosis: a biomechanical analysis. Foot Ankle Int 2010;31(1):69–75. https://doi.org/10.3113/FAI.2010.0069.

70. Jamieson MD, Stake IK, Brady AW, et al. Anterior Inferior Tibiofibular Ligament Suture Tape Augmentation for Isolated Syndesmotic Injuries. Foot Ankle Int 2022. https://doi.org/10.1177/10711007221082933. 10711007221082932.

71. Patel NK, Chan C, Murphy CI, et al. Hybrid Fixation Restores Tibiofibular Kinematics for Early Weightbearing After Syndesmotic Injury. Orthop J Sports Med 2020;8(9). https://doi.org/10.1177/2325967120946744. 2325967120946744.

72. Patel NK, Murphy CI, Pfeiffer TR, et al. Sagittal instability with inversion is important to evaluate after syndesmosis injury and repair: a cadaveric robotic study. J Exp Orthop 2020;7(1):18. https://doi.org/10.1186/s40634-020-00234-w.

73. LaMothe JM, Baxter JR, Murphy C, et al. Three-Dimensional Analysis of Fibular Motion After Fixation of Syndesmotic Injuries With a Screw or Suture-Button Construct. Foot Ankle Int 2016;37(12):1350–6. https://doi.org/10.1177/1071100716666865.

74. Bragonzoni L, Russo A, Girolami M, et al. The distal tibiofibular syndesmosis during passive foot flexion. RSA-based study on intact, ligament injured and screw fixed cadaver specimens. Arch Orthop Trauma Surg 2006;126(5):304–8. https://doi.org/10.1007/s00402-006-0131-8.

75. Che J, Li C, Gao Z, et al. Novel anatomical reconstruction of distal tibiofibular ligaments restores syndesmotic biomechanics. Knee Surg Sports Traumatol Arthrosc 2017;25(6):1866–72. https://doi.org/10.1007/s00167-017-4485-y.

76. Wu R, Wu H, Arola D, et al. Real-time three-dimensional digital image correlation for biomedical applications. J Biomed Opt 2016;21(10):107003. https://doi.org/10.1117/1.JBO.21.10.107003.

77. Pang EQ, Bedigrew K, Palanca A, et al. Ankle joint contact loads and displacement in syndesmosis injuries repaired with Tightropes compared with screw fixation in a static model. Injury 2019;50(11):1901–7. https://doi.org/10.1016/j.injury.2019.09.012.

78. Soin SP, Knight TA, Dinah AF, et al. Suture-button versus screw fixation in a syndesmosis rupture model: a biomechanical comparison. Foot Ankle Int 2009;30(4):346–52. https://doi.org/10.3113/FAI.2009.0346.

79. Seyhan M, Donmez F, Mahirogullari M, et al. Comparison of screw fixation with elastic fixation methods in the treatment of syndesmosis injuries in ankle fractures. Injury 2015;46(Suppl 2):S19–23. https://doi.org/10.1016/j.injury.2015.05.027.

80. Nelson OA. Examination and repair of the AITFL in transmalleolar fractures. J Orthop Trauma 2006;20(9):637–43. https://doi.org/10.1097/01.bot.0000211145.08543.4a.

81. Shoji H, Teramoto A, Sakakibara Y, et al. Kinematics and Laxity of the Ankle Joint in Anatomic and Nonanatomic Anterior Talofibular Ligament Repair: A Biomechanical Cadaveric Study. Am J Sports Med 2019;47(3):667–73. https://doi.org/10.1177/0363546518820527.

82. Wood AR, Arshad SA, Kim H, et al. Kinematic Analysis of Combined Suture-Button and Suture Anchor Augment Constructs for Ankle Syndesmosis Injuries. Foot Ankle Int 2020;41(4):463–72. https://doi.org/10.1177/1071100719898181.

83. Kelly M, Vasconcellos D, Osman WS, et al. Alterations in tibiotalar joint reaction force following syndesmotic injury are restored with static syndesmotic fixation. Clin Biomech (Bristol, Avon) 2019;69:156–63. https://doi.org/10.1016/j.clinbiomech.2019.07.013.

84. Goetz JE, Rungprai C, Rudert MJ, et al. Screw fixation of the syndesmosis alters joint contact characteristics in an axially loaded cadaveric model. Foot Ankle Surg 2019;25(5):594–600. https://doi.org/10.1016/j.fas.2018.05.003.

85. Gräff P, Alanazi S, Alazzawi S, et al. Screw fixation for syndesmotic injury is stronger and provides more contact area of the joint surface than TightRope®:

A biomechanical study. Technol Health Care 2020;28(5):533–9. https://doi.org/
10.3233/THC-191638.

86. Markolf KL, Jackson SR, McAllister DR. Syndesmosis fixation using dual 3.5 mm
and 4.5 mm screws with tricortical and quadricortical purchase: a biomechanical study. Foot Ankle Int 2013;34(5):734–9. https://doi.org/10.1177/
1071100713478923.

87 Hansen M, Le L, Wertheimer S, et al. Syndesmosis fixation: analysis of shear
stress via axial load on 3.5-mm and 4.5-mm quadricortical syndesmotic screws.
J Foot Ankle Surg 2006;45(2):65–9. https://doi.org/10.1053/j.jfas.2005.12.004.

88. Pereira DS, Koval KJ, Resnick RB, et al. Tibiotalar contact area and pressure
distribution: the effect of mortise widening and syndesmosis fixation. Foot Ankle
Int 1996;17(5):269–74. https://doi.org/10.1177/107110079601700506.

89. Bai L, Zhang W, Guan S, et al. Syndesmotic malreduction may decrease fixation
stability: a biomechanical study. J Orthop Surg Res 2020;15:64. https://doi.org/
10.1186/s13018-020-01584-y.

90. Vasarhelyi A, Lubitz J, Zeh A, et al. [Dynamic gait analysis of blocked distal tibiofibular joint following syndesmotic complex lesions]. Z Orthop Unfall 2009;
147(4):439–44. https://doi.org/10.1055/s-0029-1185695.

91. Taskesen A, Okkaoglu MC, Demirkale I, et al. Dynamic and Stabilometric Analysis After Syndesmosis Injuries. J Am Podiatr Med Assoc 2020;110(4). https://
doi.org/10.7547/18-174. Article_9.

92. Alastuey-López D, Seral B, Pérez MÁ. Biomechanical evaluation of syndesmotic
fixation techniques via finite element analysis: Screw vs. suture button. Comput
Methods Programs Biomed 2021;208:106272. https://doi.org/10.1016/j.cmpb.
2021.106272.

93. Hamid KS, Scott AT, Nwachukwu BU, et al. The Role of Fluid Dynamics in
Distributing Ankle Stresses in Anatomic and Injured States. Foot Ankle Int
2016;37(12):1343–9. https://doi.org/10.1177/1071100716660823.

94. Li H, Chen Y, Qiang M, et al. Computational biomechanical analysis of postoperative inferior tibiofibular syndesmosis: a modified modeling method. Comput
Methods Biomech Biomed Engin 2018;21(5):427–35. https://doi.org/10.1080/
10255842.2018.1472770.

95. Liacouras PC, Wayne JS. Computational modeling to predict mechanical function of joints: application to the lower leg with simulation of two cadaver studies.
J Biomech Eng 2007;129(6):811–7. https://doi.org/10.1115/1.2800763.

96. Liu Q, Zhang K, Zhuang Y, et al. Analysis of the stress and displacement distribution of inferior tibiofibular syndesmosis injuries repaired with screw fixation: a
finite element study. PLoS One 2013;8(12):e80236. https://doi.org/10.1371/
journal.pone.0080236.

97. Liu Q, Zhao G, Yu B, et al. Effects of inferior tibiofibular syndesmosis injury and
screw stabilization on motion of the ankle: a finite element study. Knee Surg
Sports Traumatol Arthrosc 2016;24(4):1228–35. https://doi.org/10.1007/
s00167-014-3320-y.

98. Vance NG, Vance RC, Chandler WT, et al. Can Syndesmosis Screws Displace
the Distal Fibula? Foot Ankle Spec 2021;14(3):201–5. https://doi.org/10.1177/
1938640020912092.

99. Verim O, Er MS, Altinel L, et al. Biomechanical evaluation of syndesmotic screw
position: a finite-element analysis. J Orthop Trauma 2014;28(4):210–5. https://
doi.org/10.1097/BOT.0b013e3182a6df0a.

100. Wei F, Braman JE, Weaver BT, et al. Determination of dynamic ankle ligament
strains from a computational model driven by motion analysis based kinematic

data. J Biomech 2011;44(15):2636–41. https://doi.org/10.1016/j.jbiomech.2011.08.010.

101. Zhu ZJ, Zhu Y, Liu JF, et al. Posterolateral ankle ligament injuries affect ankle stability: a finite element study. BMC Musculoskelet Disord 2016;17:96. https://doi.org/10.1186/s12891-016-0954-6.

102. Mercan N, Yıldırım A, Dere Y. Biomechanical Analysis of Tibiofibular Syndesmosis Injury Fixation Methods: A Finite Element Analysis. J Foot Ankle Surg 2022. https://doi.org/10.1053/j.jfas.2022.05.007.

103. Er MS, Verim O, Altinel L, et al. Three-dimensional finite element analysis used to compare six different methods of syndesmosis fixation with 3.5- or 4.5-mm titanium screws: a biomechanical study. J Am Podiatr Med Assoc 2013;103(3):174–80. https://doi.org/10.7547/1030174.

104. Er MS, Verim O, Eroglu M, et al. Biomechanical evaluation of syndesmotic screw design via finite element analysis and Taguchi's method. J Am Podiatr Med Assoc 2015;105(1):14–21. https://doi.org/10.7547/8750-7315-105.1.14.

105. Hariri AE, Mirzabozorg H, Esmaeili R, et al. Predicting ankle joint syndesmotic screw lifetime using finite element and fatigue analysis. J Orthopaedics, Trauma Rehabil 2022;29(1). https://doi.org/10.1177/22104917221077274. 221049172210772.

106. Scranton PE, McMaster JG, Kelly E. Dynamic fibular function: a new concept. Clin Orthop Relat Res 1976;118:76–81.

Reflections on Presurgical and Postsurgical Gait Mechanics After 50 Years of Total Ankle Arthroplasty and Perspectives on the Next Decade of Advancement

Robin M. Queen, PhD[a,b,*], Daniel Schmitt, PhD[c]

KEYWORDS

- Total ankle replacement • Gait • Recovery

KEY POINTS

- Total ankle arthroplasty has high patient satisfaction as a result of pain reduction, improvements in walking speed, and greater ankle dorsiflexion, which provide a relatively fast and stable step after surgery.
- Total ankle arthroplasty does not restore gait, especially in the push-off phase, to level experiences by age-matched persons without arthritis.
- Future studies should examine aspects of the push-off phase and total body mechanics to further explore the systemic impacts of total ankle arthroplasty on gait efficiency.

 Video content accompanies this article at http://www.foot.theclinics.com.

INTRODUCTION

As we approach the 50th anniversary of total ankle replacement, it is time to take a look at what we have learned about walking mechanics before and after total ankle arthroplasty (TAA). The ankle was the last major lower extremity joint to be treated with replacement.[1,2] The first ankle arthroplasty was attempted in 1970,[3] and then

[a] Department of Biomedical Engineering and Mechanics, Kevin P. Granata Biomechanics Lab, Blacksburg, VA, USA; [b] Department of Orthopaedic Surgery, Virginia Tech Carilion School of Medicine, Roanoke, VA, USA; [c] Department of Evolutionary Anthropology, Duke University, Durham, NC 27708, USA
* Corresponding author. Virginia Tech, 495 Old Turner Street, 300 Norris Hall, Blacksburg, VA 24061.
E-mail address: rmqueen@vt.edu

Foot Ankle Clin N Am 28 (2023) 99–113
https://doi.org/10.1016/j.fcl.2022.10.005
1083-7515/23/© 2022 Elsevier Inc. All rights reserved.

many more were performed between 1972 and 1981 with generally poor outcomes.[4–8] It is worth noting at the outset that there is a rich literature on this topic and more recently on gait mechanics and ankle replacement. It is beyond the scope of this article to cite all the interesting work that exists. We have decided to highlight useful and exemplary articles that we hope will inspire the reader to explore further and we apologize to anyone who was omitted.

Early arthroplasty failed to restore healthy gait and often these early devices could not survive long without requiring a revision procedure. As a result, until the late 1980s fusion (arthrodesis) was favored over replacement (arthroplasty), and in most cases, arthrodesis is still the most common surgical choice.[9] In the late 1990s papers began arguing forcefully that arthroplasty was a safe, effective, and durable intervention across age groups and should be used instead of fusion.[10] However, even today, TAA is not used universally accepted as the primary surgical intervention for the treatment of ankle arthritis and data on the effect of TAA on gait mechanics remained limited (see Ref,[9] for a review).

Since the turn of this century, there has been a great deal of development of new implants ranging from relatively simple fixed-bearing models to mobile-bearing models with a lot of discussion about their relative efficacy.[11–18] As will be detailed below, many papers focus on key factors like patient-reported outcome scores that assess pain, disability, overall patient satisfaction, and the need for surgical revision, all of which we recognize as important outcome measures.

Fewer papers, however, address remaining questions of whether TAA restores what might be considered healthy (non-arthritic) gait, irrespective of decreases in pain and increases in activity and walking speed. In this area—ankle biomechanics—data have been consistent and somewhat limited in its findings. As we try to digest what we know after 50 years, there is a need for a comprehensive summary of what we know and what the next steps need to be to evaluate the effectiveness of TAA as an intervention for ankle arthritis. Here, we describe the current state of research (with selected though not exhaustive references) and current thought on the biomechanical effectiveness of TAA as an intervention. Based on these data, we take a position on the value of TAA and what we need to know to continue improving patient outcomes. It is hoped that this inspires further discussion and research in this area.

With this goal in mind, we review surgical approaches to ankle arthritis and ask the question: does joint replacement simply relieve pain or do these interventions restore normal ankle and foot function? This question may seem surprising given the overwhelmingly positive patient and surgeon satisfaction following TAA.[10,14,15] It is often assumed that interventions that increase patient activity and have high satisfaction achieve those goals by restoring normal function. This may be the case, but little data exist to support that assumption.

With the intention of providing a critical review of the current state of knowledge about TAA and gait mechanics, we explore the biomechanics of the ankle before and after surgery to assess the effectiveness of this intervention. At a minimum, TAA serves as effective pain relief,[9,15,19] and patients generally report high satisfaction with surgery, regardless of implant type.[10,12–15,20,21] Therefore, TAA allows patients to move with less pain, which could explain mobility improvements. Little evidence exists that supports the belief that TAA completely restores ankle function. All the studies described later in this review show that certain aspects of gait and foot mechanics—walking speed, step length, peak dorsiflexion, and center of pressure (COP) position—do improve, other aspects—plantarflexion, costs of locomotion, and ground reaction force profiles—do not. Although restoration of normal ankle function is not essential for the completion of activities of daily living, altered biomechanics that persist after TAA can lead to a need for revision of the implant, overloading of the unaffected limb, and poor movement mechanics of unaffected joints on the ipsilateral and contralateral limbs. The determination of these impacts along with an assessment of the energetic costs of locomotion need to be a central focus of future research in this area.

BIOMECHANICS OF THE HUMAN FOOT AND ANKLE
Spatiotemporal Values

Humans walk with a striding gait on relatively stiff limbs and complete a heel-to-toe progression with each step.[22] During human locomotion, there is a period where the foot is in contact with the ground (stance phase) and a period when the foot is not in contact with the ground, and foot and leg are moved forward and positioned for the next heel strike (swing phase) (**Fig. 1**). During swing, the hip and knee must flex and the ankle must dorsiflex to clear the ground and position the heel to contact the ground at the initiation of the subsequent support (stance) phase (see **Fig. 1**). Humans progress from heel-to-toe during stance phase of each foot and we alternate left and right contacts. As a result, during each stride, there is a period of single support and a period of double support. The length of double support depends on walking speed, with the double support phase being shorter as walking speed increases. Patients with arthritis have changes in these spatiotemporal variables—walking speed, step length, stride length, and stance phase duration—which can be corrected by fusion and to a greater extent by replacement.[23–25]

Range of Motion

The human ankle must be able to move freely in dorsiflexion and plantarflexion and serve several roles including (1) being as a stable landing point for each step, (2) acting to absorb shock as load (both impact and continuous) is applied, and finally (3) serving as a rigid lever to propel the body forward. The ankle joints (talocrural and subtalar) are central to those functions. Without a mobile ankle that can dorsiflex during the swing phase, at heel strike, and during most of support phase, a stable heel-to-toe gait pattern would be impossible. This is evident in individuals with limited ankle motion, ankle fusion, or loss of anterior calf muscle function (who land flat on their foot, have foot drop, or exhibit a marching gait pattern that in turn raises metabolic costs of locomotion).[26] During the support phase of gait, it is critical that there is an effective heel-to-toe progression,[22] which is initiated at heel strike by placing the center of pressure below the heel (**Fig. 2A and B**). The COP then moves forward and crosses from lateral to medial ending at the distal hallux during toe-off (see **Fig. 2A and B**). Starting with midsupport, the foot and its compressed arch must form a rigid lever and progress to a powerful toe-off with the center of pressure between digits 1 and 2 and a high load on the hallux (see **Fig. 2A and B**). As midsupport progresses, the heel leaves the ground, and the ankle remains dorsiflexed, but progresses toward plantarflexion for toe-off.

These foot postures are reflected both in the movement of the COP and in the movements of the whole body (**Fig. 3**). The human leg can be modeled as a loaded spring like a shock absorber with mass concentrated at one end.[27] In the simplest walking gait models, a foot and ankle are not included and the knee functions as the spring, with the amount of angular change during stance relative to force applied representing the spring stiffness. A foot can be added and is well modeled as a semicircle to reflect heel-to-toe progression. In a normal walking step with a stiff limb (limited joint collapse; a stiff spring), the center of mass (COM) rises from a low position at heel

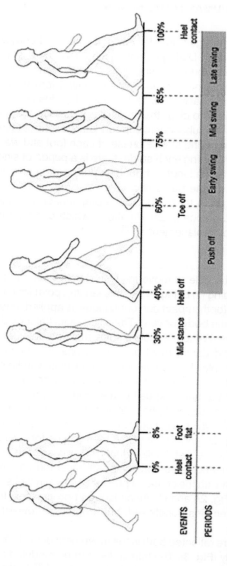

Fig. 1. Phases of the gait cycle in normal human locomotion. Note the dorsiflexed position of the ankle to permit a stable landing at heel contact and the relatively plantarflexed position as the body is driven forward from heel-off to toe-off.

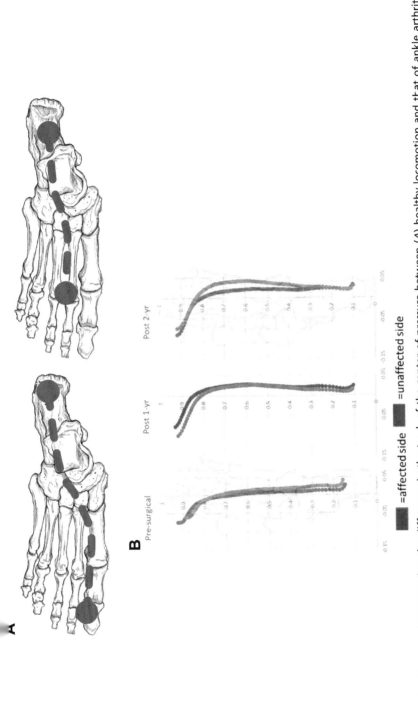

Fig. 2. Foot images demonstrating the difference in the track of the center of pressure between (A) healthy locomotion and that of ankle arthritis patients. In the former, the COP travels from heel to distal digit I. In the latter, the COP begins more distally in the hindfoot and ends more proximally between digits I and II. (B) The effect of TAA on COP pathways in the affected (blue) and unaffected (brown) sides before surgery and 1 and 2 years after surgery. At both time points, the COM begins in a more normal position relative to the heel and end in a more normal position relative to the hallux on both the affected and unaffected sides.

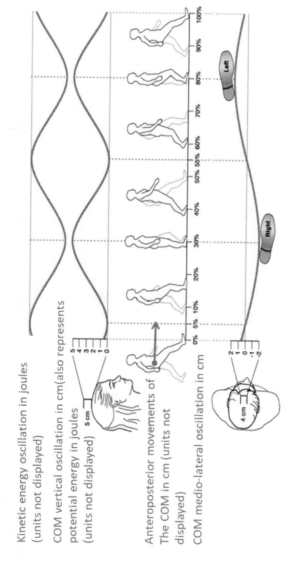

Kinetic energy oscillation in joules (units not displayed)

COM vertical oscillation in cm(also represents potential energy in joules (units not displayed)

Anteroposterior movements of The COM in cm (units not displayed)

COM medio-lateral oscillation in cm

Fig. 3. The trajectory of the center of mass (COM) during normal, healthy walking in vertical and mediolateral directions. The vertical movements of the COM fluctuate, with the low point at heel strike and the high point at midstance; these can be used to calculate the gravitational potential energy (GPE) of the COM throughout the step. The velocity of these fluctuations can be calculated and used to calculate vertical kinetic energy (KE). Anteroposterior COM movements can be used to calculate COM forward velocity and KE. Mediolateral movements of the COM also fluctuate with each footfall and can be used to calculate mediolateral COM velocity and KE. Those three kinetic energies can be summed as modeled in the top curve. If PE and KE are out of phase and of the same magnitude, high amounts of PE energy will be converted into KE and reduce the muscular work required to accelerate the COM. KE is highest at the propulsive phase of gait. Changes in plantar flexion will change both the timing and magnitude of KE and reduce energy recovery.

strike to a high position at midstance (see **Fig. 3**). In this arrangement, the gravitational potential energy (PE) at midstance is highest and that PE, derived from the vertical movements of the COM, is converted to kinetic energy (KE), derived from velocities of the COM in all three planes, as the pendulum falls again, allowing the COM to move upward and forward at the next heel strike (see **Fig. 3**). As a result, the energy of the COM is converted back into PE (see **Fig. 3**). In a functioning system, the paths of PE and KE of the COM are the same amplitude and shape and out of phase (incongruent) yielding about 70% energy recovery.[28,29] This recovery reduces muscular work needed to accelerate the COM.

In addition to this pendular exchange pattern, a substantial amount of work is required when the COM is redirected from generally downward to generally upward during the step-to-step transition, described as the time between heel strike of one limb and toe-off of the other during walking.[30,31] It is thought that the change in COM velocity during this period is achieved through angular changes in its path, where the size of the angles is influenced by step length, stride length, and the duration of the double support phase. It has been suggested that muscular work associated with this change in the COM velocity is a significant contributor to the energetic cost of walking. One way to moderate collisional costs is to extend double support time so that two limbs are in contact with the ground during the collision and to have complete heel-to-toe progression with the COP under the foot, in such a way that the foot can be modeled as a curved structure providing a "rolling foot."[22] These two issues—energy recovery and COM collisions—have profound implications for muscular work and both mechanisms can be disrupted by limits in joint motion associated with arthritis. This is a relatively new area of research that will be discussed more below and deserves further investigation as we strive to improve mechanical outcomes for patients.

THE EFFECT OF UNTREATED ANKLE ARTHRITIS ON GAIT MECHANICS

The devastating effects of ankle arthritis on people who experience it is well understood and described in the literature.[17,32,33] Sufferers often do not seek medical intervention in the early stages of the disease, which may be due to the fact that ankle arthritis is less common than arthritis in the knee, hip, and hands, and patients are not always aware of their options.[34–36] Ankle arthritis is most often the result of overuse/overloading from ankle sprains and ligament tears as well as from trauma such as fractures and avascular necrosis or previous ankle surgery.[33,35] Ankle arthritis has profound patient-reported impacts, with some studies having reported that ankle arthritis can be as physically and emotionally debilitating as end-stage renal disease, congestive heart failure, and chronic low back pain.[32,33,37] This pain can lead to inactivity, weight gain, and further disease progression, as well as resulting in gait changes that can lead to altered mechanics at the affected joints resulting in compensatory mechanics of other joints on the ipsilateral and contralateral sides and to overloading and under-loading of various joints in the lower limbs. TAA, which is steadily replacing fusion as the standard of care, can relieve the disability associated with ankle arthritis by aligning the ankle joint and the foot in a way that results in improved gait mechanics allowing patients to move effectively and with less pain.[1,2,9,11,15,17,19,23,24,38]

Gait mechanics in arthritis patients are substantially influenced by limits in range of motion and by pain associated with joint loading. Sagittal plane motion (dorsiflexion and plantarflexion) is the primary plane of motion addressed throughout this review. Although we also address, though to a lesser degree, with inversion and eversion and the associated mediolateral movements of the COP. Healthy gait progresses from heel strike at the most proximal part of the foot through toe-off at the distal portions of digits I and II. To accomplish this heel-to-toe progression, a patient must be able to maintain stable dorsiflexion. Without that the patient adopts a flat-footed marching gait during which the COP remains relatively distal. During push-off, the foot must move out of dorsiflexion (<90) and into plantarflexion to drive the body forward. Without this shift, patients will have incomplete COP progression, reduced power, and will adopt a vertical lift toe-off using the hip and knee and as a result will take smaller steps.

Patterns of loading are distinct for patients with ankle OA in which they reduce loads on the affected leg and increase those on the unaffected (**Fig. 4**).[9,19,38,39] Key time points of high load are (1) at heel contact (impact and rapid loading; heel contact in **Fig. 1** and impact spike in **Fig. 4**B), (2) during weight acceptance (foot flat in **Fig. 1** and first peak of the ground reaction force in **Fig. 4**B), and (3) during the propulsive phase (period between heel-off and toe-off in **Fig. 1** and the second peak of the ground reaction force in **Fig. 4**). With each step, those loading peaks can be one to two times body weight. To experience healthy loading, the foot must move through its full normal range of motion to land on the heel with the foot in a dorsiflexed position and to push-off from the toes as the ankle becomes more plantarflexed (see **Figs. 1** and **3**).

BIOMECHANICS OF PRESURGICAL, END-STAGE ANKLE ARTHRITIS

Ankle arthritis is painful and makes walking tiring.[25,40,41] Before intervention, patients with ankle arthritis tire easily and are often limited in their capabilities to carry out activities of daily living.[25,40] Some of the fatigue associated with arthritis may be the result of increased heart rate and respiratory rate.[40] Patients with arthritis experience inhibited gait with slower walking speed, reduced range of motion, lower ground reaction forces, and potentially higher locomotor costs associated with lower recovery.[9,11,19,23–25,32,37,39,41–46] Examining these parameters sets the stage for the question of does TAA restore function.

All studies to date show that arthritis patients have reduced walking speed and smaller step lengths.[9,11,19,23–25,32,37,39,41–46] They also show spatiotemporal asymmetry,[44] with the less affected limb compensating for loss of function in the affected limb.[19,23,43] Consistently, patients with ankle arthritis are shown to have reduced range of motion with reduced dorsiflexion and plantarflexion.[19,23,43] This leaves patients with a limited ability to complete a healthy heel-to-toe progression, specifically limiting the ability to push-off effectively, a deficiency compensated for at the hip and to a lesser extent the knee.[9] In association with this pattern, presurgical patients show a reduced COP progression, a pattern that is also asymmetric between limbs.[47]

Peak forces are lower and lack the characteristic two peaks that are present during normal walking, reflecting changes in COM movement.[28] In a comprehensive study of unilateral hip, knee, and ankle arthritis patients, after controlling for walking speed, it was found that ankle arthritis patients have shorter strides, longer double support phases, and slower walking speeds (the former two being associated with gait speed). In addition, patients with ankle arthritis had noticeably altered force traces with flattened ground reaction force curves that essentially lacked the two typical peaks of weight acceptance and propulsion[39] (see **Fig. 4**).

Directly related to the decreased walking speed, limited plantarflexion, flattened ground reaction forces, and changes in whole body movements are the exchange of PE and KE (recovery) pattern that typifies human locomotion (see **Fig. 3**).[41] Independent studies have shown that patients with ankle arthritis had lower energy recovery values[41,46] indicating that they did not fully exchange PE and KE during locomotion.

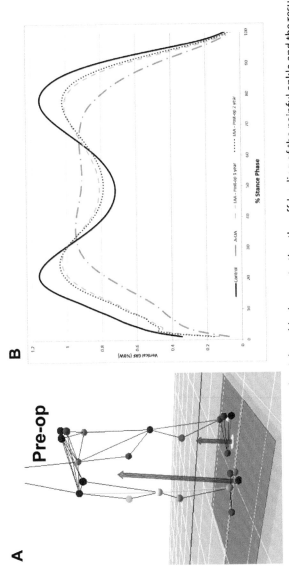

Fig. 4. (*A*) Representative patient with ankle arthritis in the right ankle demonstrating the off-loading of the painful ankle and the resulting increase in ground reaction forces on the contralateral limb. The larger red arrow represents a higher resultant ground reaction force on the unaffected leg. Also see supplementary videos. (*B*) Representative vertical force traces from asymptomatic adult human age-matched controls (*solid line*) compared with preoperative ankle arthritis patients (*dashed-dotted orange line*), and those patients at one (*dashed blue*) and 2 years (*dotted purple line*) after surgery. Note the low values (as seen in *A* of this figure as well) and flattened curve with no clear weight acceptance and propulsive peaks. TAA restored the shape, though not the magnitude, of vertical force curves and maintained those values and shape for at least 2 years.

Queen and colleagues speculated that this reflected the lack of plantarflexion and full extension of the COP to the hallux, leading to an early and incomplete push-off.[46] This was supported a study that demonstrated that ankle arthritis patients have a COP that does not move completely from heel to toe.[47] The study of Zeininger and colleagues revealed that the COP began more distally (in front of the heel) and did not progress as far proximally (behind the distal part of the hallux) when compared with a control group suggesting that heel-to-toe progression is incomplete in patients with ankle arthritis.[47]

When explored holistically, untreated ankle arthritis leads to altered kinematics at the ankle as well as throughout the lower extremity, which could lead to the reported increase in energetic costs of locomotion. The increase in energetic costs could lead to the inactivity reported in these patients and highlight the need for effective treatment to return biomechanics to those more closely approximating healthy gait.

Surgical Intervention Effectiveness

There are two phases of TAA development in the past 50 years. The first is the early period (the first 25 years) where simple devices were being explored as an option. The second is the current period in which more sophisticated long-lasting devices are being used. The current treatment options for end-stage ankle arthritis include ankle arthrodesis (eg, a fusion), TAA, and total ankle distraction arthroplasty. Arthrodesis was the state-of-the-art solution for ankle arthritis even into the late 1990s.[1,2,9] During the intervening quarter of a century, it has been shown that TAA can effectively reduce pain based on patient self-report.[10,15] However, it seems that the function of the ankle after TAA continues to remain deficient, with ankle range of motion remaining similar to what is present before TAA surgery.[9,19,48] The disparity between a patient's perceived surgical success (eg, decreased pain and increased quality of life) and the mechanical performance of their ankle makes it difficult to determine which parameters are the most important in determining postoperative success. For example, patients with less pain may increase their activity, but, ultimately, this increased activity could lead to disease progression in other joints (eg, the hips, knees, and contralateral ankle) secondary to poor gait mechanics and loading asymmetries. In addition, some patients may achieve pain relief from their TAA, but still find that moving is fatiguing.

Ankle fusion versus total ankle arthroplasty

For a long time, ankle arthrodesis (fusion of ankle bones) was the standard surgical treatment for end-stage ankle arthritis; however, the association between arthrodesis and ipsilateral adjacent joint degeneration, as well as persistent functional limitations due to its elimination of ankle motion, has driven the development and widespread use of TAA as an alternative.[1,2,8] TAA implants have been designed to return and maintain to some degree functional levels of ankle joint mobility that is not available in fusion, and overall receives positive patient scores following TAA. Although limited studies on the effectiveness of TAA combined with surgeon habit preference as well as patient needs and resource limitations have meant that fusion remains a common treatment.[9] Multiple studies have addressed clinical outcomes, radiographic alignment, and survival rates of ankle implants.[1] Only recently have researchers explored changes in gait mechanics associated with TAA and specifically different implant types. For instance, it has been shown that the range of motion measured with a goniometer,[16,49] gait speed, stride length, ground reaction forces, peak planar flexion moment, and maximum ankle dorsiflexion all increase after TAA,[23,24,42,43,49] however, peak plantarflexion and plantarflexion moment (all those and Queen) does not improve nor are costs of locomotion reduced.[25] The limited findings of improvement following TAA are consistent and often last 2 years and some even persist for 5 years, though there is also decline in many other measures.[9]

However, even 50 years after the first TAA was performed, the question remains as to how effective TAA is for patients compared with fusion. Based on published literature, ankle arthroplasty decreases pain and increases walking speed, step length, and stride length,[15,19,24,49] however, these improvements do not last, with some decline between the first year and the second year following surgery.[9] In addition, improvements in spatiotemporal variables do not come with a change in peak plantarflexion or peak plantarflexion moment[9,19,38] or changes in power or mechanical loading.[24,25] In addition, patients with an arthrodesis that are converted to a TAA have worse outcomes that those with a primary TAA and continue to have limited ankle range of motion compared with primary ankle replacement patients.[38]

Total ankle arthroplasty outcomes compared with presurgical ankle arthritis

The results for gait mechanics following TAA when compared with presurgical mechanics are similar to the studies described above when comparing TAA gait mechanics to fusion. Following TAA, patients walk faster and have longer step lengths[9,11,17,19,21,23,24,38,43,47,48] as well as having improved dorsiflexion, while plantarflexion remains unchanged following surgery (Video 1). In addition, Doets and colleagues[25,41] have shown no improvements in power or energy consumption, though Detrembleur and Leemrijse showed some improvement in energetic cost. The area of energetic cost remains an area that deserves further exploration.

Total ankle arthroplasty outcomes based on implant type

There has been considerable discussion over the past 25 years regarding implant design.[1,2] Two major classes of implants have been developed: mobile- and fixed-bearing. The degree to which these implants improve outcomes is understudied and remains an area of research and debate.[9] Most TAA studies use a single implant for comparison with ankle fusion. Fewer studies[9,21] have examined multiple implant types in the same study. Studies have produced relatively small or no differences in gait. One previous study demonstrated moderate variations in the clinical outcomes between the two implant classes,[20] whereas another, which was a randomized controlled trial, demonstrated no statistical difference between the fixed-bearing and mobile-bearing[21] implants when examining joint kinematics or kinetics. Overall, there seems to be little difference between fixed- and mobile-bearing prosthesis and even less difference between types of mobile-bearing prostheses when examining gait mechanics. Although it is worth noting that controlled studies in which surgeons randomized the implant used are rare and difficult to conduct. This is an area ripe for further study with the proper experimental design. As an example, Queen and colleagues performed a randomized control trial, rare as surgeons resist randomization in surgical approaches that show limited differences between fixed- and mobile-bearing implants.[21]

In addition to the range of motion described above, TAA has the potential to improve symmetry and COP progression. Gait asymmetries are common in patients with arthritis[44,48] and in TAA populations and they persist following surgery.[48] The variables that remain asymmetric following TAA include the vertical ground reaction force and peak plantarflexion angle.[48] In addition, asymmetry in the COP trajectory remains following TAA with the affected limb having a shorter stance time and total path length.[47] Given these outcomes it is clear that surgical interventions for ankle arthritis, especially TAA, are effective relative to being left untreated. In addition, the changes seen in the first year following TAA do not always remaining when assessing these patients more than 2 years following surgery.

NEXT STEPS

Fifty years after the first ankle replacement surgeries were performed a lot has been learned and we still have much to explore with regarding to changing joint replacements and questions of clinical significance and outcome improvements. Primary and secondary ankle arthritis interventions can be evaluated using simple measures of physical performance such as walking speed. However, with the advent of more easily accessible biomechanics tools and video analysis methods that can be used in clinical settings,[50] clinicians will be able to evaluate gait mechanics including spatiotemporal variables, limb symmetry, ankle motion, forces, moments, and even measures of energy costs to improve walking gait and postoperative recovery. Ankle mechanics variables that can be easily examined in these settings include spatiotemporal measures like walking speed, step length, stance time, and swing time as well as more precise measures including peak forces and the shape of these curves (which are surrogates for whole body motion and energy costs) and plantarflexion angle which reflect joint motion and power production. Areas that demand further attention are energetic costs of locomotion, power production, and limb asymmetry. In addition, questions regarding the development and use of standardized postoperative rehabilitation will be essential for improving functional outcomes.

SUMMARY

TAA is the state-of-the-art surgical intervention for ankle arthritis. This is a surgical procedure with high patient satisfaction in part because of the immense pain-relief patients' experience. TAA results in improved patient satisfaction and in some cases mobility improvements when compared with nonsurgical treatment and arthrodesis. Based on current knowledge, there is no reason to believe that implant type drives outcomes or that one implant is superior when assessing gait restoration. All implant types provide pain relief and some changes in walking speed, energy costs, and COP movement, yet no improvements in plantarflexion or plantarflexion power. Clearly pain relief and concomitant improvements in walking speed and patient activity are not enough to restore normal gait. Patients are still walking abnormally and overloading other joints in the ipsilateral and contralateral limbs up to 2 years after surgery. Additional therapeutic interventions are necessary to restore function and improve walking efficiency.

CLINICS CARE POINTS

- Total ankle arthroplasty should be considered an acceptable standard of care for severe ankle arthritis.
- Gait assessment with a focus on gait speed and gait stability should be added to presurgical and postsurgical care to assess recovery.
- Postoperative care should focus on improving the push-off phase of walking.

DISCLOSURE

The authors have no conflicts to disclose.

SUPPLEMENTARY DATA

Supplementary data related to this article can be found online at https://doi.org/10.1016/j.fcl.2022.10.005.

REFERENCES

1. Vickerstaff JA, Miles AW, Cunningham JL. A brief history of total ankle replacement and a review of the current status. Med Eng Phys 2007;29(10):1056–64.
2. Bonasia DE, Dettoni F, Femino JE, et al. Total ankle replacement: why, when and how? Iowa orthopaedic J 2010;30:119.
3. Lord G, Marotte J. Total ankle prosthesis. Technic and 1st results. Apropos of 12 cases. Revue de chirurgie orthopédique et réparatrice de l'appareil moteur. 1973;59(2):139–51.
4. Lachiewicz P, Inglis A, Ranawat C. Total ankle replacement in rheumatoid arthritis. J Bone Joint Surg Am 1984;66(3):340–3.
5. Bolton-Maggs B, Sudlow R, Freeman M. Total ankle arthroplasty. A long-term review of the London Hospital experience. J Bone Joint Surg Br 1985;67(5):785–90.
6. Unger AS, Inglis AE, Mow CS, et al. Total ankle arthroplasty in rheumatoid arthritis: a long-term follow-up study. Foot & Ankle 1988;8(4):173–9.
7. Kitaoka HB, Patzer GL. Clinical results of the Mayo total ankle arthroplasty. JBJS 1996;78(11):1658–64.
8. Henne TD, Anderson JG. Total ankle arthroplasty: a historical perspective. Foot Ankle Clin 2002;7(4):695–702.
9. Queen R. Directing clinical care using lower extremity biomechanics in patients with ankle osteoarthritis and ankle arthroplasty. J Orthopaedic Res 2017;35(11):2345–55.
10. Kofoed H, Lundberg-Jensen A. Ankle arthroplasty in patients younger and older than 50 years: a prospective series with long-term follow-up. Foot Ankle Int 1999;20(8):501–6.
11. Mazur JM, Schwartz E, Simon SR. Ankle arthrodesis. Long-term follow-up with gait analysis. J bone Jt Surg Am volume 1979;61(7):964–75.
12. Wood P, Deakin S. Total ankle replacement: the results in 200 ankles. J bone Jt Surg Br 2003;85(3):334–41.
13. Wood P, Karski M, Watmough P. Total ankle replacement: the results of 100 mobility total ankle replacements. J Bone Jt Surg Br 2010;92(7):958–62.
14. Wood P, Prem H, Sutton C. Total ankle replacement: medium-term results in 200 Scandinavian total ankle replacements. J Bone Jt Surg Br volume 2008;90(5):605–9.
15. Knecht SI, Estin M, Callaghan JJ, et al. The Agility total ankle arthroplasty: seven to sixteen-year follow-up. JBJS 2004;86(6):1161–71.
16. Buechel Sr FF, Buechel FF Jr, Pappas MJ Jr. Ten-year evaluation of cementless Buechel-Pappas meniscal bearing total ankle replacement. Foot Ankle Int 2003;24(6):462–72.
17. Valderrabano V, Nigg BM, von Tscharner V, et al. Gait analysis in ankle osteoarthritis and total ankle replacement. Clin Biomech 2007;22(8):894–904.
18. Barg A, Phisitkul P, Saltzman C. Mobile-vs. fixed-bearing total ankle prostheses: A systematic review and meta-analysis. Foot & Ankle Orthopaedics 2017;2(3). 2473011417S2473000108.
19. Queen RM, De Biasio JC, Butler RJ, et al. Changes in pain, function, and gait mechanics two years following total ankle arthroplasty performed with two modern fixed-bearing prostheses. Foot Ankle Int 2012;33(7):535–42.

20. Valderrabano V, Pagenstert GI, Müller AM, et al. Mobile-and fixed-bearing total ankle prostheses: is there really a difference? Foot Ankle Clin 2012;17(4):565–85.

21. Queen RM, Franck CT, Schmitt D, et al. Are there differences in gait mechanics in patients with a fixed versus mobile bearing total ankle arthroplasty? A randomized trial. Clin Orthopaedics Relat Research. 2017;475(10):2599–606.

22. Kuo AD. The six determinants of gait and the inverted pendulum analogy: A dynamic walking perspective. Hum Move Sci 2007;26(4):617–56.

23. Singer S, Klejman S, Pinsker E, et al. Ankle arthroplasty and ankle arthrodesis: gait analysis compared with normal controls. JBJS 2013;95(24):e191.

24. Doets HC, Middelkoop Mv, Houdijk H, et al. Gait analysis after successful mobile bearing total ankle replacement. Foot Ankle Int 2007;28(3):313–22.

25. Doets HC, Vergouw D, Veeger HD, et al. Metabolic cost and mechanical work for the step-to-step transition in walking after successful total ankle arthroplasty. Hum Move Sci 2009;28(6):786–97.

26. Fowler PT, Botte MJ, Mathewson JW, et al. Energy cost of ambulation with different methods of foot and ankle immobilization. J orthopaedic Res 1993; 11(3):416–21.

27. Geyer H, Seyfarth A, Blickhan R. Compliant leg behaviour explains basic dynamics of walking and running. Proc R Soc B: Biol Sci 2006;273(1603):2861–7.

28. Cavagna GA, Heglund NC, Taylor CR. Mechanical work in terrestrial locomotion: two basic mechanisms for minimizing energy expenditure. Am J Physiology-Regulatory, Integr Comp Physiol 1977;233(5):R243–61.

29. Griffin TM, Roberts TJ, Kram R. Metabolic cost of generating muscular force in human walking: insights from load-carrying and speed experiments. J Appl Physiol 2003;95(1):172–83.

30. Ruina A, Bertram JE, Srinivasan M. A collisional model of the energetic cost of support work qualitatively explains leg sequencing in walking and galloping, pseudo-elastic leg behavior in running and the walk-to-run transition. J Theor Biol 2005;237(2):170–92.

31. Lee DV, Comanescu TN, Butcher MT, et al. A comparative collision-based analysis of human gait. Proc R Soc B: Biol Sci 2013;280(1771):20131779.

32. Agel J, Coetzee JC, Sangeorzan BJ, et al. Functional limitations of patients with end-stage ankle arthrosis. Foot Ankle Int 2005;26(7):537–9.

33. Thomas RH, Daniels TR. Ankle Arthritis. JBJS 2003;85(5):923–36.

34. Huch K, Kuettner KE, Dieppe P. Osteoarthritis in ankle and knee joints. Paper presented at: Seminars in arthritis and rheumatism1997.

35. Saltzman CL, Salamon ML, Blanchard GM, et al. Epidemiology of ankle arthritis: report of a consecutive series of 639 patients from a tertiary orthopaedic center. Iowa orthopaedic J 2005;25:44.

36. Brown TD, Johnston RC, Saltzman CL, et al. Posttraumatic osteoarthritis: a first estimate of incidence, prevalence, and burden of disease. J orthopaedic Trauma 2006;20(10):739–44.

37. Segal AD, Shofer J, Hahn ME, et al. Functional limitations associated with end-stage ankle arthritis. JBJS 2012;94(9):777–83.

38. Queen RM, Sparling TL, Butler RJ, et al. Patient-reported outcomes, function, and gait mechanics after fixed and mobile-bearing total ankle replacement. JBJS 2014;96(12):987–93.

39. Schmitt D, Vap A, Queen RM. Effect of end-stage hip, knee, and ankle osteoarthritis on walking mechanics. Gait & posture 2015;42(3):373–9.

40. Waters R, Barnes G, Husserl T, et al. Comparable energy expenditure after arthrodesis of the hip and ankle. J Bone Joint Surg Am Volume 1988;70(7): 1032–7.
41. Detrembleur C, Leemrijse T. The effects of total ankle replacement on gait disability: analysis of energetic and mechanical variables. Gait & posture 2009; 29(2):270–4.
42. Dyrby C, Chou LB, Andriacchi TP, et al. Functional evaluation of the Scandinavian total ankle replacement. Foot Ankle Int 2004;25(6):377–81.
43. Flavin R, Coleman SC, Tenenbaum S, et al. Comparison of gait after total ankle arthroplasty and ankle arthrodesis. Foot Ankle Int 2013;34(10):1340–8.
44. Hughes-Oliver C, Srinivasan D, Schmitt D, et al. Gender and limb differences in temporal gait parameters and gait variability in ankle osteoarthritis. Gait & Posture 2018;65:228–33.
45. Muir DC, Amendola A, Saltzman CL. Long-term outcome of ankle arthrodesis. Foot Ankle Clin 2002;7(4):703–8.
46. Queen RM, Sparling TL, Schmitt D. Hip, knee, and ankle osteoarthritis negatively affects mechanical energy exchange. Clin Orthopaedics Relat Research 2016; 474(9):2055–63.
47. Zeininger A, Schmitt D, Hughes-Oliver C, et al. The effect of ankle osteoarthritis and total ankle arthroplasty on center of pressure position. J Orthopaedic Research. 2021;39(6):1245–52.
48. Queen RM, Butler RJ, Adams SB Jr, et al. Bilateral differences in gait mechanics following total ankle replacement: a two year longitudinal study. Clin Biomech 2014;29(4):418–22.
49. Doets HC, Brand R, Nelissen RG. Total ankle arthroplasty in inflammatory joint disease with use of two mobile-bearing designs. JBJS 2006;88(6):1272–84.
50. Peebles AT, Carroll MM, Socha JJ, et al. Validity of using automated two-dimensional video analysis to measure continuous sagittal plane running kinematics. Ann Biomed Eng 2021;49(1):455–68.

Definitions and Measurements of Hindfoot Alignment and Their Biomechanical and Clinical Implications

Sorin Siegler, PhD*, Luigi Piarulli, MSc, Jordan Stolle, MSc

KEYWORDS

- Hindfoot • Ankle • Subtalar • Alignment • Standards • Imaging

KEY POINTS

- Defining and measuring hindfoot, ankle, and subtalar alignment is important for current clinical applications such as total ankle replacement alignment and deformity correction.
- Three-dimensional (3D) alignment measures are gaining in popularity because cheaper, more accurate, and more accessible 3D imaging tools are available.
- Three-dimensional alignment measures are more accurate and more reliable than their two-dimensional (2D) counterparts. However, they are harder and more time consuming to obtain, more expensive, and less accessible at the present.
- Acceptable standards for hindfoot alignment (HA) are desirable. However, different standards may be required for different clinical and biomechanical applications.
- Cone beam technology used in weight-bearing CT is gaining in clinical popularity as a tool for obtaining functional, accurate 3D imaging data required for defining and measuring HA.

INTRODUCTION

Alignment, in the context of anatomical joints, is defined as the relative position and orientation between the articulating bones. Accordingly, ankle alignment (AA), subtalar alignment (SA), and hindfoot alignment (HA) indicate the relative position and orientation between the talus and tibia, calcaneus and talus, and calcaneus and tibia, respectively.[1] Various pathologic conditions and their treatment may affect AA, SA, and HA.

Department of Mechanical Engineering, Drexel University, 3141 Chestnut Street, Philadelphia, PA, USA
* Corresponding author.
E-mail address: sieglers@drexel.edu

Foot Ankle Clin N Am 28 (2023) 115–128
https://doi.org/10.1016/j.fcl.2022.11.002

Such pathologic conditions include the presence of arthritis,[2-7] severe and chronic ligament injuries, varus/valgus deformities,[2-5,8-11] and various tendon injuries such as posterior tibial tendon dysfunction[12-14] or foot bone lesions.[15]

Many of the previously mentioned pathologic conditions are accompanied by or directly cause misalignment of AA, SA, or HA. Treatments of these pathologic conditions often involve efforts to restore normal alignment in the afflicted joints. To achieve this, pretreatment and posttreatment alignment measurements are essential in order to determine the degree of misalignment present before treatment, as well as to determine whether the misalignment has been successfully remedied.[16-33] For example, image-based surgical planning in total ankle replacement (TAR) provides detailed information not only on the sizing and optimal locations of the implant but also on the degree of presurgical misalignment present and the amount of correction required to restore normal alignment.[34] In the same way, AA, SA, and HA are necessary for the evaluation of the effect of corrective osteotomies.[34,35] Therefore, for these and other diagnostic and treatment procedures, knowledge of three-dimensional (3D) normal AA, SA, and HA is essential.[36-38]

Many different methods to describe the alignment and misalignment of the hindfoot have been developed throughout the years. These methods have progressively become more precise, detailed, and accurate alongside the advancement of medical technology. Early measures of HA were often comparatively crude, relying on visual inspection and measurement of the skin surface around the ankle joint.[39-41] Natural evolutions of these measurements involved the placement of markers on key locations on the skin, the positions of which were captured by cameras in order to quantify the joint motion. Detection of the position of surface skin markers through various types of kinematic capturing systems[42-44] can provide 3D measurements of HA as well as measures of the kinematics of the hindfoot during activities such as walking or running. Such methods are limited, however, by inaccuracies introduced by relative motion between the skin and the underlying bone. Such markers are also unable to record information regarding the AA and SA because external skin markers are unable to record the position and motion of the talus.[7]

More modern measures of alignment use a variety of imaging methods, such as 2D x-ray imaging,[16,17,21,22,25-27,29,34,35,45-51] as well as 3D standard CT and MRI imaging,[39,52-54] weight-bearing cone-beam CT (WBCT) imaging,[11,20,23,28,55-65] and dual fluoroscopy.[21,66-68]

One of the most popular 2D measures of HA is the hindfoot moment arm. This measure of HA is derived from HA view, which is a coronal plane view of the hindfoot. The hindfoot moment arm is defined by measuring the horizontal distance between a line representing the weight-bearing axis of the tibia and the plantar-most aspect of the calcaneus. The weight-bearing axis of the tibia is defined by the bisection of the tibia 10 and 15 cm above the distal tibial plafond.[69]

Another 2D measure of HA is the HA angle. This angle is defined by the tibial principal axis and the calcaneal tuberosity axis. The tibial principal axis is defined in the same manner as the weight-bearing axis of the hindfoot moment arm; that is, by the bisection of the tibia 10 and 15 cm above the distal tibial plafond. The calcaneal axis is determined by the bisection of 2 transversals between lines drawn along the lateral and medial osseous contours of the calcaneus. This method considers only the posterior aspect of the calcaneus.[70]

The kite angle, also referred to as the talocalcaneal angle, relates the talus and the calcaneus, and is drawn in the transverse plane. Kite angle is defined as the angle between the longitudinal axis of the talar head and neck and the line tangent to the lateral side of the calcaneus.[45,71,72]

The talar declination angle and the calcaneal inclination angle are also considered in diagnosing hindfoot pathologic condition. Both 2D measurements are examined within a sagittal view of the hindfoot. The talar declination angle is defined as the angle between the base of support and the longitudinal axis of the head and neck of the talus. The calcaneal inclination angle is defined as the angle between the base of support and the line tangent to the planar aspect of the calcaneus. Both measures, although correlated with certain hindfoot pathologic conditions, are not pure measures of HA because they measure a bone of the hindfoot's relative position to an external position, namely the base of support.[73]

The above 2D measures are each drawn from measurements performed on 2D conventional radiographs taken at different orientations. Such measures are clinically popular because of their simplicity and ease of acquisition. These measures, however, are limited in scope because they examine the ankle in only one 2D cross section, and each captures a single angle within that 2D cross section. For this reason, only partial information on one of HA, SA, or AA is ascertained by a given measure, and the others are not included.[31,74]

Conventional CT and MRI provide 3D information on the bones and their relative position, reducing the error associated with projection planes present in 2D systems. However, they do not describe the relative bone position and orientation during a functional activity such as standing. For instance, before the introduction of the WBCT in clinical practice, HA was computed with measurements obtained without body weight from standard CT or MR images.[75] Other studies tried to simulate the body weight in standard CT leading to an applied load that varied between 10% and 50% of the physiological body weight using specialized custom loading systems.[76–78]

Three-dimensional measures performed during weight-bearing such as WBCT that are not limited to 2D projections are desirable for their ability to describe HA, SA, and AA alignment both completely and functionally. An early example of such a measurement is the foot ankle offset (FAO). This measure is determined by relating the centermost and superior most point of the talus to the line connecting the distalmost points of the calcaneus and the midpoint of the points connecting the first and fifth metatarsal heads (**Fig. 1**).[37] Although the FAO is shown to correlate to HA and can be used to

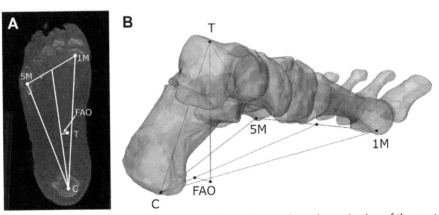

Fig. 1. The FAO is determined by the perpendicular distance from the projection of the most superior and central point of the talus onto the floor (T) with the line connecting the most distal points of the calcaneus (C) and the midpoint of the points connecting the first (1M) and fifth (5M) metatarsal heads. (*Data from* Lintz, F., et al., 3D Biometrics for Hindfoot Alignment Using Weightbearing CT. Foot Ankle Int, 2017. 38(6): p. 684-689.)

classify ankles into normal ankles, those with varus deformity, and those with valgus deformity, it is not purely a measure of HA because it incorporates the forefoot into its calculation.[9,30,38,79]

Recently, efforts are being invested in converting alignment measures that were previously taken in 2D to 3D. Measures mentioned earlier, such as the HA angle, are calculated using WBCT to construct and calculate angles between 3D axes instead of the projected angles used in 2 dimensions.[55,80,81] It has been shown that such 3D measurements, even though they maintain identical or similar definition, produce results with higher reliability than their 2D counterparts.[7]

Complete 3D alignment measures in 6 degrees-of-freedom require defining reference frames for the tibia, talus, and calcaneus. These reference frames are based entirely on the morphology and landmarks of the specific bone for which the reference frame is constructed, independent of any neighboring morphology or structure (**Fig. 2**). The relative positions of these reference frames are determined in 3 dimensions, with their relative positions of the tibia, talus, and calcaneal reference frames fully defining the alignment of the HA, SA, and AA.[55,80,82–84]

DISCUSSION

The definition and measurements of HA are crucial in clinical practice and in biomechanical research. Clinically, assessment of HA is necessary to quantify foot and ankle

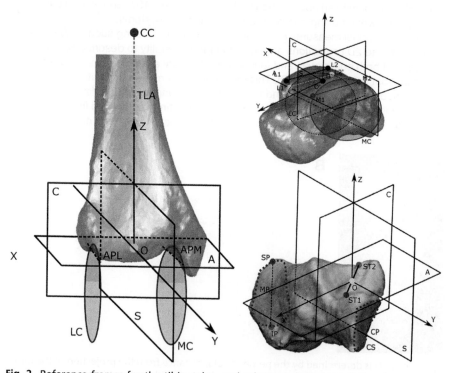

Fig. 2. Reference frames for the tibia, talus, and calcaneus used for defining the 3D alignment at the hindfoot, the ankle, and the subtalar joints. (*Data from* Stolle, J., et al., Three-dimensional ankle, subtalar, and hindfoot alignment of the normal, weightbearing hindfoot, in bilateral posture. J Orthop Res, 2022.40(10): p. 2430-2439.)

deformities and their level of severity. They can guide treatment selection and evaluation.[2,4–7,9–11,13,16–22,25–30,32,33,85,86] HA quantification is also necessary for planning surgeries such as TAR,[53,82,87–92] osteotomies for hindfoot realignment,[93–97] soft tissue reconstructions, contraction releases, or ligament repair.[8,13,16,19,26,66,92,98–102] Additionally, interoperative fluoroscopy[103,104] and HA guides can help the surgeon directly intraoperatively.[105]

In biomechanical research, defining and quantifying HA is necessary to study the effect of misalignments on load transfer and stresses on the natural interfaces across joints [9,148] or on bone-implant interfaces, such as in TAR.[53,66,82,87,101,106,107] Knowledge of these loads and stresses obtained through modeling or in-vitro studies[89,108–110] are important for the development of new surgical realignment techniques. In addition, the same parameters used to define alignment are often used for measuring the kinematics of the ankle during functional performance such as walking or running.[88,111–113] Finally, quantification of the alignment and misalignment of the HA, AA, and SA may provide an insight on the interdependence between hip and knee alignment and HA as well as on the interdependence of the alignment of joint of the foot and HA, for example, the effect of HA, AA, and SA misalignments and misalignment at the joints of the midfoot and forefoot.[48,50,92,98,99,114–125]

Historically, clinical practice relied on assessing alignment from radiographic 2D measurements. Such measures may provide a quick, convenient, and economical assessment of hindfoot deformities. Therefore, these measures continue to be popular in today's modern clinical practice.[16,17,21,25,27,29,35,45–47,49–51,87,126]

Other traditional clinical measurements of HA are performed directly on the skin with markers and goniometers. However, these are often associated with low reliability that result from large errors and lack of acceptable repeatability.[39–41]

Two-dimensional images represent the projection of 3D structures on a specific plane (sagittal, coronal, or axial), where different inclinations of the x-ray beam and superposition of the bones can distort the morphology,[55,115,127] making 2D measurements prone to error.[30,60,128] In contrast, alignment measurements based on 3D imaging have the potential of eliminating this problem, resulting in better reliability.[38,45,58,129]

Measurements relying on 3D imaging have the potential of providing more in depth and accurate assessment of HA.[31,74] These can be used for a variety of clinical applications such as customized implants and surgical planning.[82,83] However, many of these measures obtained from 3D image acquisition such as the CT, MRI, dual fluoroscopy, are expensive and time consuming. Deriving these alignment parameters typically requires segmentation, 3D rendering, and sophisticated analysis software compared with their corresponding 2D counterparts.[55,80,83,89,110,111,130]

Alignment of AA, HA, and SA is most likely strongly influenced by the loads applied to the foot. This fact has been recognized by clinicians for many decades, resulting in many of them relying on weight-bearing x-ray imaging for alignment assessment.[21,24,29,49,126,129,131–134] The presence of loading, such as body weight, allows the computation of the functional HA, showing the morphological distribution of the bones during daily routine activities, such as standing.[121] However, it is not clear what level of weight-bearing is needed to obtain a functional assessment of HA.[135] For instance, 2 studies found a high correlation between non–weight-bearing and weight-bearing 3D HA parameters.[36,59] Other studies showed that HA in pathological cases should be performed under body weight to avoid an underestimation of the severity of the deformity.[6,30,57,77,78,134]

In general, it is shown that HA measurements computed on weight-bearing 3D images better represent the severity of osseous derangement.[28,52,55,57,80] Earlier it was claimed that 3D alignment measurements are time consuming, requiring manual or semiautomatic imaging processing. Although in general this is true, one outstanding exception is the FAO, a 3D weight-bearing HA measurement that is currently gaining clinical popularity.[30,37,38,79,136]

Three-dimensional–based alignment measurements are currently gaining in popularity because more clinicians realize that they provide more meaningful and objective measurements of hindfoot deformities. However, certain bottlenecks exist, and these prevent the rapid adoption of these measurements in the clinic. Some of the most critical obstacles include (1) The time-consuming nature of obtaining these measurements with image segmentation being the most time consuming. This recognized problem has resulted in many past and present efforts in automating the image segmentation process[83,137]; (2) The lack of current acceptable standards for alignment parameters, without which communication between clinicians and researcher is difficult. Although the need for widely acceptable standards is well recognized, standards should not be applied rigidly across disciplines and clinical applications, and it should be recognized that different clinical or biomechanical applications may require different alignment standards. For example, the parameters required for optimal alignment of TAR may be different from the standards required for aligning the ankle using ligament reconstruction, or from prescribing in-shoe orthotics to correct foot deformity such as a valgus or varus deformity; (3) High cost of 3D imaging compared with their 2D counterparts, as well as the reluctance of clinicians to accept novel and unfamiliar measurements to which they are not accustomed. Clearly the cost of 3D imaging is quickly decreasing. However, the cost gap between 3D and 2D imaging is still wide. In addition, clinicians who are familiar with 2D imaging having much experience interpreting those images are hard press to abandon, or even supplement, those immediate and readily available measurements with more complicated, less immediate, and less accessible measurement, which may be harder to interpret and may require additional extensive training.

SUMMARY

This article presents a critical review of the past and the current state of the art in defining and measuring hindfoot, ankle, and SA. It describes the transition occurring at present from 2D to 3D alignment measurements, which accompany the emergence of new, functional, high-resolution imaging modalities such as the WBCT. The transition to 3D measurements is clinically difficult for various reasons including time, cost, and ease of interpretation. However, these highly accurate and detailed alignment parameters help in the development of new clinical surgical approaches such as personalized surgical tools and surgical implants and as such are expected to continue to thrive and gain in popularity. It is expected that in the near future both 2D and 3D measures of alignment will continue to coexist particularly in clinical practice. To ease and enhance the transition and acceptability of 3D alignment measurements, new acceptable standards for different clinical application are highly desirable.

CLINICS CARE POINTS

- When evaluating HA, evaluate and chose among the many available measures and standards the one most appropriate for the specific clinical application.
- For nonurgent clinical applications, such as deformity correction or fitting of TARs, an accurate and complete 3D alignment assessment is advisable and sometimes necessary.

> • If available and feasible, rely on weight-bearing CT for evaluating HA. It emerges as a superior 3D alternative to 2D functional assessments measures such as weight-bearing x-ray imaging.

DISCLOSURE

The authors have nothing to disclose.

REFERENCES

1. Wu G, Siegler S, Allard P, et al. ISB recommendation on definitions of joint coordinate system of various joints for the reporting of human joint motion–part I: ankle, hip, and spine. International Society of Biomechanics. J Biomech 2002; 35(4):543–8.
2. Bernasconi A, Najefi AA, Goldberg AJ. Comparison of mechanical axis of the limb versus anatomical axis of the tibia for assessment of tibiotalar alignment in end-stage ankle arthritis. Foot Ankle Int 2021;42(5):616–23.
3. Knupp M, Stufkens S, van Bergen C, et al. Effect of supramalleolar varus and valgus deformities on the tibiotalar joint: a cadaveric study. Foot Ankle Int 2011;32(6):609–15.
4. Liu H, Sugamoto K, Itohara T, et al. In vivo three-dimensional skeletal alignment analysis of the hindfoot valgus deformity in patients with rheumatoid arthritis. J Orthop Res 2007;25(3):330–9.
5. Mitsui H, Hirano T, Yui A, et al. Relations of ankle alignment and MRI findings of ankle osteoarthritis. Foot Ankle Orthopaedics 2017;2(3).
6. Barg A, Pagenstert G, Hügle T, et al. Ankle osteoarthritis: etiology, diagnostics, and classification. Foot Ankle Clin 2013;18(3):411–26.
7. Kvarda P, Heisler L, Krähenbühl N, et al. 3D assessment in posttraumatic ankle osteoarthritis. Foot Ankle Int 2021;42(2):200–14.
8. Lee GW, Wang SH, Lee KB. Comparison of intermediate to long-term outcomes of total ankle arthroplasty in ankles with preoperative varus, valgus, and neutral alignment. J Bone Joint Surg Am 2018;100(10):835–42.
9. Lintz F, Bernasconi A, Mehdi N, et al. Weightbearing CT Analysis of Hindfoot Alignment in Chronic Lateral Ankle Instability: a Multivariate Analysis of 124 Feet. Foot Ankle Orthopaedics 2017;2(3).
10. Van Bergeyk AB, Younger A, Carson B. CT analysis of hindfoot alignment in chronic lateral ankle instability. Foot Ankle Int 2002;23(1):37–42.
11. Lintz F, Bernasconi A, Baschet L, et al. Relationship Between Chronic Lateral Ankle Instability and Hindfoot Varus Using Weight-Bearing Cone Beam Computed Tomography. Foot Ankle Int 2019;40(10):1175–81.
12. Mann RA, Thompson FM. Rupture of the posterior tibial tendon causing flat foot. Surgical treatment. J Bone Joint Surg Am 1985;67(4):556–61.
13. Sturbois-Nachef N, Allart E, Grauwin MY, et al. Tibialis posterior transfer for foot drop due to central causes: Long-term hindfoot alignment. Orthop Traumatol Surg Res 2019;105(1):153–8.
14. Zhang Y, Xu J, Wang X, et al. An in vivo study of hindfoot 3D kinetics in stage II posterior tibial tendon dysfunction (PTTD) flatfoot based on weight-bearing CT scan. Bone Joint Res 2013;2(12):255–63.
15. Paul J, Hinterwimmer S, Vavken P, et al. [Association between Hindfoot Alignment and Localisation of Osteochondral Lesions of the Talus]. Z Orthop Unfall 2014;152(4):389–92.

16. Arangio G, Rogman A, Reed JF 3rd. Hindfoot alignment valgus moment arm increases in adult flatfoot with Achilles tendon contracture. Foot Ankle Int 2009; 30(11):1078–82.

17. Arunakul M, Amendola A, Gao Y, et al. Tripod index: a new radiographic parameter assessing foot alignment. Foot Ankle Int 2013;34(10):1411–20.

18. Baverel L, Brilhault J, Odri G, et al. Influence of lower limb rotation on hindfoot alignment using a conventional two-dimensional radiographic technique. Foot Ankle Surg 2017;23(1):44–9.

19. Benedetti MG, Berti L, Straudi S, et al. Clinicoradiographic assessment of flexible flatfoot in children. J Am Podiatr Med Assoc 2010;100(6):463–71.

20. de Cesar Netto C, Bernasconi A, Roberts L, et al. Foot alignment in symptomatic national basketball association players using weightbearing cone beam computed tomography. Orthop J Sports Med 2019;7(2). 2325967119826081.

21. Hastings MK, Sinacore DR, Mercer-Bolton N, et al. Precision of foot alignment measures in Charcot arthropathy. Foot Ankle Int 2011;32(9):867–72.

22. Iyengar KP, Azzopardi CA, Fitzpatrick J, et al. Calcaneal offset index to measure hindfoot alignment in pes planus. Skeletal Radiol 2022;51(8):1631–7.

23. Bernasconi A, Cooper L, Lyle S, et al. Intraobserver and interobserver reliability of cone beam weightbearing semi-automatic three-dimensional measurements in symptomatic pes cavovarus. Foot Ankle Surg 2020;26(5):564–72.

24. Burssens A, Peeters J, Buedts K, et al. Measuring hindfoot alignment in weight bearing CT: a novel clinical relevant measurement method. Foot Ankle Surg 2016;22(4):233–8.

25. Lamm BM, Mendicino RW, Catanzariti AR, et al. Static rearfoot alignment: a comparison of clinical and radiographic measures. J Am Podiatr Med Assoc 2005;95(1):26–33.

26. Lamm BM, Stasko PA, Gesheff MG, et al. Normal foot and ankle radiographic angles, measurements, and reference points. J Foot Ankle Surg 2016;55(5): 991–8.

27. Lee J, Lee HS, Kim JW, et al. Radiographic parameters of the normal ankle syndesmosis: Comparison between hindfoot alignment view and anteroposterior view. J Int Med Res 2022;50(5). 3000605221098862.

28. Lobo CFT, Pires EA, Bordalo-Rodrigues M, et al. Imaging of progressive collapsing foot deformity with emphasis on the role of weightbearing cone beam CT. Skeletal Radiol 2022;51(6):1127–41.

29. Robinson I, Dyson R, Halson-Brown S. Reliability of clinical and radiographic measurement of rearfoot alignment in a patient population. The Foot 2001; 11(1):2–9.

30. Rojas EO, Barbachan Mansur NS, Dibbern K, et al. Weightbearing computed tomography for assessment of foot and ankle deformities: the iowa experience. Iowa Orthop J 2021;41(1):111–9.

31. Sutter R, Pfirrmann CW, Espinosa N, et al. Three-dimensional hindfoot alignment measurements based on biplanar radiographs: comparison with standard radiographic measurements. Skeletal Radiol 2013;42(4):493–8.

32. Wang B, Saltzman CL, Chalayon O, et al. Does the subtalar joint compensate for ankle malalignment in end-stage ankle arthritis? Clin Orthop Relat Res 2015; 473(1):318–25.

33. Tuijthof GJ, Herder JL, Scholten PE, et al. Measuring alignment of the hindfoot. J Biomech Eng 2004;126(3):357–62.

34. Neri T, Barthelemy R, Tourne Y. Radiologic analysis of hindfoot alignment: comparison of Meary, long axial, and hindfoot alignment views. Orthop Traumatol Surg Res 2017;103(8):1211–6.
35. Reilingh ML, Beimers L, Tuijthof GJM, et al. Measuring hindfoot alignment radiographically: the long axial view is more reliable than the hindfoot alignment view. Skeletal Radiol 2010;39(11):1103–8.
36. Haldar A, Bernasconi A, Junaid SE, et al. 3D imaging for hindfoot alignment assessment: a comparative study between non-weight-bearing MRI and weight-bearing CT. Skeletal Radiol 2021;50(1):179–88.
37. Lintz F, Welck M, Bernasconi A, et al. 3D Biometrics for Hindfoot Alignment Using Weightbearing CT. Foot Ankle Int 2017;38(6):684–9.
38. Zhang JZ, Lintz F, Bernasconi A, et al. 3D Biometrics for hindfoot alignment using weightbearing computed tomography. Foot Ankle Int 2019;40(6):720–6.
39. Haight HJ, Dahm DL, Smith J, et al. Measuring standing hindfoot alignment: reliability of goniometric and visual measurements. Arch Phys Med Rehabil 2005; 86(3):571–5.
40. Ohnishi T, Hida M, Nagasaki T, et al. Reliability of laser-assisted hindfoot alignment evaluation. J Phys Ther Sci 2020;32(1):38–41.
41. Ohnishi T, Hida M, Nakamura Y, et al. Novel method for evaluation of hindfoot alignment in weight-bearing position using laser beam. J Phys Ther Sci 2018; 30(3):474–8.
42. Kranzl A, Karoline S, Margit G. Influence of walking speed on foot angles in healthy adults using the Oxford foot model. Gait Posture 2019;73:437–8.
43. Schallig W, van den Noort JC, McCahill J, et al. Comparing the kinematic output of the Oxford and Rizzoli Foot Models during normal gait and voluntary pathological gait in healthy adults. Gait Posture 2020;82:126–32.
44. Wright CJ, Arnold BL, Coffey TG, et al. Repeatability of the modified Oxford foot model during gait in healthy adults. Gait Posture 2011;33(1):108–12.
45. Carrara C, Caravaggi P, Belvedere C, et al. Radiographic angular measurements of the foot and ankle in weight-bearing: A literature review. Foot Ankle Surg 2020;26(5):509–17.
46. Choi JY, Lee HI, Kim JH, et al. Radiographic measurements on hindfoot alignment view in 1128 asymptomatic subjects. Foot Ankle Surg 2021;27(4):366–70.
47. Harper MC. Stress radiographs in the diagnosis of lateral instability of the ankle and hindfoot. Foot Ankle 1992;13(8):435–8.
48. Johnson TM, Hentges MJ, McMillen RL, et al. Effect of the first tarsometatarsal (modified lapidus) arthrodesis on hindfoot alignment. J Foot Ankle Surg 2021; 60(2):318–21.
49. Mendicino RW, Catanzariti AR, John S, et al. Long leg calcaneal axial and hindfoot alignment radiographic views for frontal plane assessment. J Am Podiatr Med Assoc 2008;98(1):75–8.
50. Tanaka Y, Takakura Y, Fujii T, et al. Hindfoot alignment of hallux valgus evaluated by a weightbearing subtalar x-ray view. Foot Ankle Int 1999;20(10):640–5.
51. Yang C, Xu X, Hu M, et al. Optimization of hindfoot alignment radiography. Acta Radiol 2017;58(6):719–25.
52. Barg A, Bailey T, Richter M, et al. Weightbearing computed tomography of the foot and ankle: emerging technology topical review. Foot Ankle Int 2018;39(3): 376–86.
53. de Keijzer DR, Joling BSH, Sierevelt IN, et al. Influence of preoperative tibiotalar alignment in the coronal plane on the survival of total ankle replacement: a systematic review. Foot Ankle Int 2020;41(2):160–9.

54. Lee JH, Rathod CM, Park H, et al. Longitudinal observation of changes in the ankle alignment and tibiofibular relationships in hereditary multiple exostoses. Diagnostics (Basel) 2020;10(10):752–65.

55. Carrara C, Belvedere C, Caravaggi P, et al. Techniques for 3D foot bone orientation angles in weight-bearing from cone-beam computed tomography. Foot Ankle Surg 2021;27(2):168–74.

56. Carrino JA, Al Muhit A, Zbijewski W, et al. Dedicated cone-beam CT system for extremity imaging. Radiology 2014;270(3):816–24.

57. de Cesar Netto C, Schon LC, Thawait GK, et al. Flexible adult acquired flatfoot deformity: comparison between weight-bearing and non-weight-bearing measurements using cone-beam computed tomography. J Bone Joint Surg Am 2017;99(18):e98.

58. de Cesar Netto C, Shakoor D, Roberts L, et al. Hindfoot alignment of adult acquired flatfoot deformity: a comparison of clinical assessment and weightbearing cone beam CT examinations. Foot Ankle Surg 2019;25(6):790–7.

59. Hamard M, Neroladaki A, Bagetakos I, et al. Accuracy of cone-beam computed tomography for syndesmosis injury diagnosis compared to conventional computed tomography. Foot Ankle Surg 2020;26(3):265–72.

60. Pilania K, Jankharia B, Monoot P. Role of the weight-bearing cone-beam CT in evaluation of flatfoot deformity. Indian J Radiol Imaging 2019;29(4):364–71.

61. Posadzy M, Desimpel J, Vanhoenacker F. Cone beam CT of the musculoskeletal system: clinical applications. Insights Imaging 2018;9(1):35–45.

62. Shakoor D, de Cesar Netto C, Thawait GK, et al. Weight-bearing radiographs and cone-beam computed tomography examinations in adult acquired flatfoot deformity. Foot Ankle Surg 2021;27(2):201–6.

63. Wachowsky MR, et al. Comparing hindfoot alignment measurement techniques in weight-bearing CT (PedCAT) in children. Foot Ankle Surg 2017;23.

64. Tuominen EK, Kankare J, Koskinen SK, et al. Weight-bearing CT imaging of the lower extremity. AJR Am J Roentgenol 2013;200(1):146–8.

65. Burssens A, Van Herzele E, Leenders T, et al. Weightbearing CT in normal hindfoot alignment - Presence of a constitutional valgus? Foot Ankle Surg 2018;24(3):213–8.

66. Berlet GC, Penner MJ, Lancianese S, et al. Total ankle arthroplasty accuracy and reproducibility using preoperative CT scan-derived, patient-specific guides. Foot Ankle Int 2014;35(7):665–76.

67. Tsukeoka T, Tsuneizumi Y, Lee TH. Accuracy of the second metatarsal as a landmark for the extramedullary tibial cutting guide in total knee arthroplasty. Knee Surg Sports Traumatol Arthrosc 2014;22(12):2969–74.

68. Nosewicz TL, Knupp M, Bolliger L, et al. The reliability and validity of radiographic measurements for determining the three-dimensional position of the talus in varus and valgus osteoarthritic ankles. Skeletal Radiol 2012;41(12):1567–73.

69. Saltzman CL, el-Khoury GY. The hindfoot alignment view. Foot Ankle Int 1995;16(9):572–6.

70. Williamson ER, Chan JY, Burket JC, et al. New radiographic parameter assessing hindfoot alignment in stage II adult-acquired flatfoot deformity. Foot Ankle Int 2015;36(4):417–23.

71. Ippolito E, Fraracci L, Farsetti P, et al. Validity of the anteroposterior talocalcaneal angle to assess congenital clubfoot correction. AJR Am J Roentgenol 2004;182(5):1279–82.

72. Masquijo JJ, Tourn D, Torres-Gomez A. Reliability of the talocalcaneal angle for the evaluation of hindfoot alignment. Rev Esp Cir Ortop Traumatol (Engl Ed 2019;63(1):20–3.

73. Meyr AJ, Sansosti LE, Ali S. A pictorial review of reconstructive foot and ankle surgery: evaluation and intervention of the flatfoot deformity. J Radiol Case Rep 2017;11(6):26–36.

74. Leardini A, Durante S, Belvedere C, et al. Weight-bearing CT Technology in Musculoskeletal Pathologies of the Lower Limbs: Techniques, Initial Applications, and Preliminary Combinations with Gait-Analysis Measurements at the Istituto Ortopedico Rizzoli. Semin Musculoskelet Radiol 2019;23(6):643–56.

75. Buck FM, Hoffmann A, Mamisch-Saupe N, et al. Diagnostic performance of MRI measurements to assess hindfoot malalignment. An assessment of four measurement techniques. Eur Radiol 2013;23(9):2594–601.

76. Kido M, Ikoma K, Imai K, et al. Load response of the tarsal bones in patients with flatfoot deformity: in vivo 3D study. Foot Ankle Int 2011;32(11):1017–22.

77. Ferri M, Scharfenberger AV, Goplen G, et al. Weightbearing CT scan of severe flexible pes planus deformities. Foot Ankle Int 2008;29(2):199–204.

78. Hirschmann A, Pfirrmann CW, Klammer G, et al. Upright cone CT of the hindfoot: comparison of the non-weight-bearing with the upright weight-bearing position. Eur Radiol 2014;24(3):553–8.

79. Lintz F, Ricard C, Mehdi N, et al. Hindfoot alignment assessment by the foot-ankle offset: a diagnostic study. Arch Orthop Trauma Surg 2022.

80. Pavani C, Belvedere C, Ortolani M, et al. 3D measurement techniques for the hindfoot alignment angle from weight-bearing CT in a clinical population. Sci Rep 2022;12(1):16900.

81. Rogati G, Leardini A, Ortolani M, et al. Semi-automatic measurements of foot morphological parameters from 3D plantar foot scans. J Foot Ankle Res 2021; 14(1):18.

82. Belvedere C, Siegler S, Fortunato A, et al. New comprehensive procedure for custom-made total ankle replacements: medical imaging, joint modeling, prosthesis design, and 3D printing. J Orthop Res 2019;37(3):760–8.

83. Ortolani M, Leardini A, Pavani C, et al. Angular and linear measurements of adult flexible flatfoot via weight-bearing CT scans and 3D bone reconstruction tools. Sci Rep 2021;11(1):16139.

84. Stolle J, Lintz F, de Cesar Netto C, et al. Three-dimensional ankle, subtalar, and hindfoot alignment of the normal, weightbearing hindfoot, in bilateral posture. J Orthop Res 2022;40(10):2430–9.

85. de Cesar Netto C, Kunas GC, Soukup D, et al. Correlation of clinical evaluation and radiographic hindfoot alignment in stage II adult-acquired flatfoot deformity. Foot Ankle Int 2018;39(7):771–9.

86. Flores DV, Mejía Gómez C, Fernández Hernando M, et al. Adult acquired flatfoot deformity: anatomy, biomechanics, staging, and imaging findings. Radiographics 2019;39(5):1437–60.

87. Barg A, Elsner A, Anderson AE, et al. The effect of three-component total ankle replacement malalignment on clinical outcome: pain relief and functional outcome in 317 consecutive patients. J Bone Joint Surg Am 2011;93(21): 1969–78.

88. Frigg A, Nigg B, Hinz L, et al. Clinical relevance of hindfoot alignment view in total ankle replacement. Foot Ankle Int 2010;31(10):871–9.

89. Kuo CC, Lu HL, Leardini A, et al. Three-dimensional computer graphics-based ankle morphometry with computerized tomography for total ankle replacement design and positioning. Clin Anat 2014;27(4):659–68.

90. Son HS, Choi JG, Ahn J, et al. Hindfoot alignment change after total ankle arthroplasty for varus osteoarthritis. Foot Ankle Int 2021;42(4):431–9.

91. Usuelli FG, Maccario C, Indino C, et al. Evaluation of hindfoot alignment after fixed- and mobile-bearing total ankle prostheses. Foot Ankle Int 2020;41(3):286–93.

92. Yamasaki Y, Maeyama A, Miyazaki K, et al. Evaluation of the hindfoot alignment before and after total knee arthroplasty. J Clin Orthop Trauma 2022;31:101947.

93. Choi JY, Cha SM, Yeom JW, et al. Effect of the additional first ray osteotomy on hindfoot alignment after calcaneal osteotomy for the correction of mild-to-moderate adult type pes plano-valgus. J Orthop Surg (Hong Kong) 2017;25(1). 2309499016684747.

94. Choi JY, Song SJ, Kim SJ, et al. Changes in Hindfoot Alignment After High or Low Tibial Osteotomy. Foot Ankle Int 2018;39(9):1097–105.

95. Lee WC, Moon JS, Lee HS, et al. Alignment of ankle and hindfoot in early stage ankle osteoarthritis. Foot Ankle Int 2011;32(7):693–9.

96. Miyazaki K, Maeyama A, Yoshimura I, et al. Influence of hindfoot alignment on postoperative lower limb alignment in medial opening wedge high tibial osteotomy. Arch Orthop Trauma Surg 2021.

97. Peiffer M, Belvedere C, Clockaerts S, et al. Three-dimensional displacement after a medializing calcaneal osteotomy in relation to the osteotomy angle and hindfoot alignment. Foot Ankle Surg 2020;26(1):78–84.

98. Burssens A, De Roos D, Barg A, et al. Alignment of the hindfoot in total knee arthroplasty: a systematic review of clinical and radiological outcomes. Bone Joint J 2021;103-B(1):87–97.

99. Butler JJ, Mercer NP, Hurley ET, et al. Alignment of the hindfoot following total knee arthroplasty: a systematic review. World J Orthop 2021;12(10):791–801.

100. Hara Y, Ikoma K, Arai Y, et al. Alteration of hindfoot alignment after total knee arthroplasty using a novel hindfoot alignment view. J Arthroplasty 2015;30(1):126–9.

101. Hintermann B, Susdorf R, Krähenbühl N, et al. Axial rotational alignment in mobile-bearing total ankle arthroplasty. Foot Ankle Int 2020;41(5):521–8.

102. Mosca M, Caravelli S, Vocale E, et al. Outcome after modified grice-green procedure (SAMBB) for arthritic acquired adult flatfoot. Foot Ankle Int 2020;41(11):1404–10.

103. Jeon J, Kim JK, Song SH, et al. Assessment of hindfoot alignment: intraoperative fluoroscopy versus standing radiograph. J Foot Ankle Surg 2022;61(3):448–51.

104. Matuszewski PE, Abbenhaus E, Chen AT, et al. The effect of rotation on intraoperative fluoroscopic evaluation of hindfoot alignment and how to help prevent error. Bull Hosp Jt Dis (2013) 2020;78(4):250–4.

105. Frigg A, Jud L, Valderrabano V. Intraoperative positioning of the hindfoot with the hindfoot alignment guide: a pilot study. Foot Ankle Int 2014;35(1):56–62.

106. Espinosa N, Walti M, Favre P, et al. Misalignment of total ankle components can induce high joint contact pressures. J Bone Joint Surg Am 2010;92(5):1179–87.

107. Queen RM, Adams SB Jr, Viens NA, et al. Differences in outcomes following total ankle replacement in patients with neutral alignment compared with tibiotalar joint malalignment. J Bone Joint Surg Am 2013;95(21):1927–34.

108. Cenni F, Leardini A, Cheli A, et al. Position of the prosthesis components in total ankle replacement and the effect on motion at the replaced joint. Int Orthop 2012;36(3):571–8.

109. Chandler JT, Moskal JT. Evaluation of knee and hindfoot alignment before and after total knee arthroplasty: a prospective analysis. J Arthroplasty 2004;19(2): 211–6.

110. Claassen L, Luedtke P, Yao D, et al. The geometrical axis of the talocrural joint-Suggestions for a new measurement of the talocrural joint axis. Foot Ankle Surg 2019;25(3):371–7.

111. Blair DJ, Barg A, Foreman KB, et al. Methodology for measurement of in vivo tibiotalar kinematics after total ankle replacement using dual fluoroscopy. Front Bioeng Biotechnol 2020;8:375–87.

112. Frigg A, Nigg B, Davis E, et al. Does alignment in the hindfoot radiograph influence dynamic foot-floor pressures in ankle and tibiotalocalcaneal fusion? Clin Orthop Relat Res 2010;468(12):3362–70.

113. Wachowsky M, D'Souza S, Wirth T, et al. O 052— Comparison of anatomical Tibia-Hindfoot-Alignment and Oxford-Foot-Model marker-set measurement in weight bearing CT - effect of adjustment in the static model. Gait Posture 2018;65:107–9.

114. Burssens ABM, Buedts K, Barg A, et al. Is lower-limb alignment associated with hindfoot deformity in the coronal plane? A weightbearing ct analysis. Clin Orthop Relat Res 2020;478(1):154–68.

115. Dagneaux L, Moroney P, Maestro M. Reliability of hindfoot alignment measurements from standard radiographs using the methods of Meary and Saltzman. Foot Ankle Surg 2019;25(2):237–41.

116. Diao N, Yu F, Yang B, et al. Association between changes in hip-knee-ankle angle and hindfoot alignment after total knee arthroplasty for varus knee osteoarthritis. BMC Musculoskelet Disord 2021;22(1):610.

117. Duggal N, Paci GM, Narain A, et al. A computer assessment of the effect of hindfoot alignment on mechanical axis deviation. Comput Methods Programs Biomed 2014;113(1):126–32.

118. Etani Y, Hirao M, Ebina K, et al. Improvement of knee alignment and function after corrective surgery for hindfoot deformity: a report of 3 cases. JBJS Case Connect 2022;12(2).

119. Hadi H, Jabal Ameli M, Bagherifard A, et al. The effect of total knee arthroplasty on hindfoot alignment in patients with severe genu varum and genu valgum. Arch Bone Jt Surg 2020;8(3):413–9.

120. Hooper J, Rozell J, Walker PS, et al. The role of the hindfoot in total knee arthroplasty alignment. Bull Hosp Jt Dis (2013) 2020;78(1):65–73.

121. Ikuta Y, Nakasa T, Fujishita H, et al. An association between excessive valgus hindfoot alignment and postural stability during single-leg standing in adolescent athletes. BMC Sports Sci Med Rehabil 2022;14(1):64.

122. Lenz AL, Strobel MA, Anderson AM, et al. Assignment of local coordinate systems and methods to calculate tibiotalar and subtalar kinematics: a systematic review. J Biomech 2021;120:110344.

123. Nakada I, Nakamura I, Juji T, et al. Correlation between knee and hindfoot alignment in patients with rheumatoid arthritis: the effects of subtalar joint destruction. Mod Rheumatol 2015;25(5):689–93.

124. Okamoto Y, Otsuki S, Jotoku T, et al. Clinical usefulness of hindfoot assessment for total knee arthroplasty: persistent post-operative hindfoot pain and alignment

in pre-existing severe knee deformity. Knee Surg Sports Traumatol Arthrosc 2017;25(8):2632–9.

125. Bakshi N, Steadman J, Philippi M, et al. Association between hindfoot alignment and first metatarsal rotation. Foot Ankle Int 2022;43(1):105–12.

126. Johnson JE, Lamdan R, Granberry WF, et al. Hindfoot coronal alignment: a modified radiographic method. Foot Ankle Int 1999;20(12):818–25.

127. Barg A, Amendola RL, Henninger HB, et al. Influence of ankle position and radiographic projection angle on measurement of supramalleolar alignment on the anteroposterior and hindfoot alignment views. Foot Ankle Int 2015; 36(11):1352–61.

128. Brandenburg LS, Siegel M, Neubauer J, et al. Measuring standing hindfoot alignment: reliability of different approaches in conventional x-ray and cone-beam CT. Arch Orthop Trauma Surg 2022;142(11):3035–43.

129. Lintz F, Beaudet P, Richardi G, et al. Weight-bearing CT in foot and ankle pathology. Orthop Traumatol Surg Res 2021;107(1S):102772.

130. Brown JA, Gale T, Anderst W. An automated method for defining anatomic coordinate systems in the hindfoot. J Biomech 2020;109:109951.

131. Foran IM, Mehraban N, Jacobsen SK, et al. Impact of coleman block test on adult hindfoot alignment assessed by clinical examination, radiography, and weight-bearing computed tomography. Foot Ankle Orthop 2020;5(3). 2473011420933264.

132. Lintz F, Barton T, Millet M, et al. Ground reaction force calcaneal offset: a new measurement of hindfoot alignment. Foot Ankle Surg 2012;18(1):9–14.

133. Richter M, Seidl B, Zech S, et al. PedCAT for 3D-imaging in standing position allows for more accurate bone position (angle) measurement than radiographs or CT. Foot Ankle Surg 2014;20(3):201–7.

134. Richter M, Zech S, Hahn S. PedCAT for radiographic 3D-Imaging in standing position. Fuß Sprunggelenk 2015;13(2):85–102.

135. Buber N, Zanetti M, Frigg A, et al. Assessment of hindfoot alignment using MRI and standing hindfoot alignment radiographs (Saltzman view). Skeletal Radiol 2018;47(1):19–24.

136. de Cesar Netto C, Bang K, Mansur NS, et al. Multiplanar semiautomatic assessment of foot and ankle offset in adult acquired flatfoot deformity. Foot Ankle Int 2020;41(7):839–48.

137. Richter M, Duerr F, Schilke R, et al. Semi-automatic software-based 3D-angular measurement for Weight-Bearing CT (WBCT) in the foot provides different angles than measurement by hand. Foot Ankle Surg 2022;28(7):919–27.

Current Challenges in Chronic Ankle Instability

Review and Perspective

Matthieu Lalevée, MD, MSc[a,b], Donald D. Anderson, PhD[c,d,e],
Jason M. Wilken, PT, PhD[f,*]

KEYWORDS

- Ankle instability • Ankle sprain • Functional • Mechanical • Risk factors

KEY POINTS

- Chronic ankle instability (CAI) often leads to disability and ankle osteoarthritis resulting in a significant long-term socioeconomic burden. The management of CAI has changed little.
- CAI, relevant to multiple fields and specialties, is commonly addressed in terms of either mechanical instability or functional impairment. Basic research is needed to foster reliable translational research encompassing both mechanical and functional aspects.
- A thorough accounting of the many risk factors for CAI is needed. The development of effective preventative and treatment strategies is contingent on understanding how and why some people develop CAI after a simple ankle sprain, whereas others do not.
- Sprain simulators assessing ankle inversion and angular inversion velocity could help diagnose and quantify CAI. Such measurements will play a role in understanding the relative importance of each risk factor in CAI.

INTRODUCTION

Injuries to the ligaments of the ankle are common and represent an important socioeconomic burden.[1] The incidence of ankle sprains is approximately 7/1000 person-years in the general population and can be as high as 45/1000 person-years in physically active people,[2] with both direct and indirect financial burden.[1] Despite the frequency and impact of ankle sprains, treatment has changed little over the

[a] CETAPS EA3832, Research Center for Sports and Athletic Activities Transformations, University of Rouen Normandy, F-76821 Mont-Saint-Aignan, France; [b] Department of Orthopedic Surgery, Rouen University Hospital, 37 Bd Gambetta, Rouen 76000, France; [c] Department of Orthopedics and Rehabilitation, The University of Iowa, Iowa City, IA 52242, USA; [d] Department of Biomedical Engineering, The University of Iowa, Iowa City, IA 52242, USA; [e] Department of Industrial and Systems Engineering, The University of Iowa, Iowa City, IA 52242, USA; [f] Department of Physical Therapy and Rehabilitation Science, The University of Iowa, 500 Newton Road, 1-249 Medical Education Building, Iowa City, IA 52242-1089, USA
* Corresponding author.
E-mail address: jason-wilken@uiowa.edu

Foot Ankle Clin N Am 28 (2023) 129–143
https://doi.org/10.1016/j.fcl.2022.11.003
1083-7515/23/© 2022 Elsevier Inc. All rights reserved.

past three decades.[3] Although many individuals successfully recover from ankle sprains, nearly one-third experience chronic ankle instability (CAI) with significant short- and long-term consequences for patients, including ankle osteoarthritis.[4]

There are several reasons that may explain why we have been unable to improve the management of ankle sprain and CAI to avoid these consequences. First, CAI is a complex multifaceted condition relevant to multiple specialties, with each working to address instability from their unique point of view.[5] For example, orthopedists and sport medicine specialists primarily focus on the mechanical aspect of CAI associated with anatomical lesions amenable to surgical treatments.[6] Conversely, physiotherapists and physiatrists primarily focus on rehabilitative interventions and fuction.[7] As a result of this siloed approach to research, few studies rigorously address both aspects together. Given its complexity, a multidisciplinary approach combining the strengths of all interested parties is essential to advance the understanding and management of CAI, encompassing both functional and mechanical aspects.[8]

Second, the mechanisms whereby some patients progress to CAI following a simple sprain, whereas others manage to cope and return to a normal life, are not well understood.[1,9] An improved understanding of why some individuals develop CAI and others are able to effectively cope would be a crucial step in the management of CAI, in particular by developing preventive care. Third, CAI involves many risk factors. The accumulation of these risk factors could explain, at least in part, the occurrence and severity of CAI. A detailed accounting of potential risk factors is needed for rigorous evaluation; however, a comprehensive accounting of the risk factors appears to be lacking.

Finally, diagnostic and measurement tools to identify and track individuals at risk of CAI, before and after an acute sprain, and to propose preventive treatments are desperately needed. Currently available tools are primarily limited to questionnaires focused on sprain history and their consequences, making preventive management impossible.

Our review aimed to detail these different aspects of CAI point-by-point to guide researchers and clinicians in their research prospects.

WHY SHOULD WE IMPROVE CHRONIC ANKLE INSTABILITY MANAGEMENT?

According to a recent systematic review by Lin and colleagues,[10] the overall prevalence of CAI after a sprain is 25%, and in otherwise healthy adolescent athletes, the prevalence of CAI is 20% following an ankle sprain.[11] Despite over one-fifth of individuals progressing to CAI, ankle sprains are still considered benign injuries by many athletes and the general population.[12] It is therefore essential to advance efforts to inform the scientific and clinical community of the deleterious effects of CAI.

Michels and colleagues[13] recently showed that 1 year after an ankle sprain, 15.8% of patients have a recurrence, 8.1% remain subjectively unstable, and 6.7% suffer from residual pain. These issues seem to persist over time. In a 6.5-year follow-up study of ankle sprains, 6% of patients were unable to maintain their occupational activities, whereas 15% could only continue their original occupation with some handicap.[14] Articular lesions are one potential source of the persistent limitations. The incidence of osteochondral lesions following an ankle sprain is between 37 and 89% in the literature.[15,16] Sugimoto and colleagues[17] arthroscopically assessed the cartilage of 99 CAI ankles, finding only 23.2% of ankles with normal cartilage, whereas all the others (76.8%) presented with cartilage damage, of which 41.4% had serious lesions.

Further, Valderrabano and colleagues[18] found a 55% history of prior ligamentous lesion from sports injuries in a study of individuals with post-traumatic ankle osteoarthritis, leading them to conclude that ankle sprains are one of the main cause of post-traumatic ankle osteoarthritis. Finally, the 2016 International Ankle Consortium stated that there is growing evidence that an important consequence of ankle sprain, and the resulting high rate of CAI, is post-traumatic ankle osteoarthritis, affecting young patients and making the majority of surgical cases of post-traumatic ankle osteoarthritis.[1]

This growing body of literature supports efforts to communicate the importance of successful management of ankle sprains. Ankle sprains and especially CAI have a direct impact on patient lives, in particular because they frequently cause articular lesions that can require surgical treatment. It is therefore essential to treat CAI before the appearance of these consequences.

FUNCTIONAL AND MECHANICAL INSTABILITY

The pathophysiological concepts pertaining to CAI are frequently divided into mechanical and functional instability.[19,20] This division could stem from background differences between specialties. On the one hand, orthopedic surgeons will look for mechanical factors such as ligament laxity or gastrocnemius tightness because their experience allows them to correct these anatomical problems.[21] On the contrary, the physical therapists or physiatrists primarily focus on functional instability and factors such as deficits in proprioception or weakness of the evertors.[22] The differing perspectives are evident in the scientific literature, with most studies only assessing mechanical or functional instability and far fewer addressing both perspectives.[5] The mechanical aspect of instability involves anatomical structures such as ligaments or bone deformities, whereas the functional aspect is rather linked to proprioceptive and neuromuscular deficits.[23]

Initially, the study of CAI focused on ligamentous laxity and its mechanical aspects was predominant until Freeman introduced the concept of functional instability represented by the persistence of symptoms following an ankle sprain.[24,25] Only considering ligamentous laxity in mechanical instability is a narrow point of view. For instance, Yoshimoto and colleagues[26] showed that the recurrence of ankle sprain after surgical ligament reconstruction is higher with varus inclination of the tibial plafond. Many other factors are likely involved in mechanical instability, such as syndesmotic injury or lack of ankle dorsiflexion.[27,28] Similarly, the functional aspect of CAI is much more than persistent symptoms after an ankle sprain, including for example impaired proprioception or muscle weakness.[29,30]

Freeman was one of the first to develop a theory linking functional and mechanical instability.[24,25] His concept was that a ligament injury, which would be the cause of mechanical instability, can also be responsible for functional instability. This is because a ligament lesion can cause partial deafferentation resulting in sensorimotor impairment, leading to functional instability of the ankle. Now over 50 years later, Hertel and colleagues[31] have proposed an updated model of CAI fully encompassing its known mechanical and functional aspects. This model includes 8 primary components: primary tissue injury, pathomechanical impairments, sensory-perceptual impairments, motor-behavioral impairments, personal factors, environmental factors, component interactions, and the spectrum of clinical outcomes. These 8 components interact through 3 so-called conjectural constructs or self-organization, perception-action, and neurosignature.

This CAI model goes beyond the mechanical and functional aspects and includes interactions between its different components and considering the whole person. The triggering factor of CAI is represented in this model by the sprain and the ligamentous injury. Once the patient has sprained his ankle, they enter a loop where these 8 components influence the occurrence of a CAI. For instance, risk factors such as the pathomechanical impairments of ligamentous laxity or restricted range of motion and the motor-behavioral impairment or muscle weakness can contribute to the development of CAI. These components interact within what they called the self-organization, which is specific to each patient and represents the control of the patient's motion which is influenced by different constraints.

The different pathological factors also interact through perception-action cycles and the neurosignature. The perception-action cycles represent what the patient perceives and what the motor response to that perception will be and the neurosignature, which is influenced by many factors like genetics and the patient's lived experience, would represent the central processing of the perception-action cycles. These three conjectural constructs are unique to each person and will determine, by interacting with the risk factors, whether the patient would experience CAI or effectively cope after a sprain. This concept effectively illustrates the influence of each risk factors on the outcome and the fact that the CAI functional and mechanical aspects must be considered together and not divided.

However, this model does not provide detailed information regarding the primary risk factors influencing the prevention or management of CAI, or their relative importance. For instance, we do not know whether ankle laxity should be considered a more important risk factor for CAI than evertor muscle weakness. Going further, we also do not know which ligaments should be considered. What they call the primary tissue injury can include damage to the anterior talofibular ligament and calcaneofibular ligament, however, syndesmotic, cervical, or deltoid ligament involvement could also influence CAI.[27,32] The model does not provide information on the importance of the accumulation of these different risk factors. It is possible that a patient with six of these risk factors is more likely to develop CAI than a patient with only 2 risk factors. Finally, risk factors may be modifiable or non-modifiable. For example, an ankle varus can be medically or surgically corrected in some individuals, whereas the patient's age cannot.

In summary, the mechanical and functional aspects of CAI are closely related. Basic research that crosses medical specialties must be carried out to then allow reliable translational research encompassing the mechanical and functional aspects of CAI.

PROGRESSION FROM ACUTE SPRAIN TO CHRONIC ANKLE INSTABILITY

Our understanding of why some patients develop CAI after an acute sprain, whereas others are able to cope and return to normal life is limited. Understanding the differences between these two groups will be a crucial step in managing CAI. Knowing a priori what pushes the patient towards instability would allow preventive care to allow more individuals to successfully cope with an ankle sprain and avoid instability.

Wikstrom and colleagues[33] define a coper as a patient who has had a severe sprain but is able to resume weight-bearing activity for at least 12 months without injury, episodes of giving way and/or feelings of instability. Comparing CAI and copers patients 1 year after sprain to controls, Doherty and colleagues[34] showed that CAI patients had a deficit in dynamic balance compared with controls and copers. In a recent systematic review, Yu and colleagues[35] concluded that CAI patients exhibit adaptive strategies (primarily hip flexion to maintain stability) when landing and increased frontal ankle displacement compared with copers. Understanding these differences could allow early detection of patients at risk of CAI after a sprain and to implement preventive care.

Donovan and colleagues[36] performed a literature review in 2012 and classified the presence of CAI impairments in 4 different domains: limited range of motion, decreased strength, impaired postural control and altered movement strategies. They have developed a rehabilitation protocol specifically designed to address these 4 different domains of impairments. This helps improve CAI management, but this does not explain the origin of the differences between individuals with CAI and copers.

As described by Hertel and colleagues,[31] ligamentous injury in an ankle sprain may trigger sensorimotor changes via inflammatory and pain mediators that would result in specific sensory-perceptual and motor-behavioral impairments. Each patient would react differently to this and some of them would develop CAI. However, many factors could influence this pathway from acute sprain to CAI. Miklovic and colleagues[37] considered that the use of Donovan and colleagues[36] above-mentioned protocol can treat a large majority of CAI patients. But they did not know whether they should apply this same protocol in early rehabilitation for acute ankle sprain. They therefore decided to carry out a review of the literature to find out whether the 4 impairments they described in CAI would be present in patients with acute and subacute ankle sprains. Their conclusion was that similar domains of impairment were present in these different groups and that their rehabilitation protocol could also be applied to acute sprains. Because these impairments are present immediately after the injury, one can wonder if some of them could have been present before the trauma and if doing prophylactic rehabilitation could have avoided the initial trauma.

There are many risk factors for ankle sprain and CAI that align with both mechanical and functional concepts. Some of them could be present even before the trauma (ie, hindfoot varus), and some of them would appear after the acute sprain. As described by Hertel and colleagues[31] all these factors interact. It is likely that the more risk factors an individual has the more likely they are to sprain their ankle and develop CAI. The ankle sprain occurrence would be an addition of one of these risk factors (ligamentous laxity), which would destabilize the patient's homeostasis and cause them to develop CAI. Therefore, the most important point would be to be acquainted of these risk factors and then to understand the relative impact of each of them in sprain and CAI occurrences. A patient could either never have sprained their ankle or present an acute sprain or become coper or develop CAI. The important point would be to monitor these risk factors to correct those that are correctable. According to this theory, it would also be possible to provide prophylactic treatment, for example in athletes to avoid a first episode of acute sprain, or to prevent a subject from developing CAI after an acute sprain.

RISK FACTORS FOR CHRONIC ANKLE INSTABILITY

To collect all the CAI risk factors currently present in the literature, we conducted a rapid review using PubMed and the keywords "ankle AND lateral AND (instability OR unstable) AND (risk factor OR predict* OR relationship)". All studies available in PubMed up to May 2022 were screened. Comparative studies and systematic reviews of comparative studies involving CAI patients (comparing CAI to controls or copers or assessing recurrence of ankle sprain after treatment) were included. Case reports, narrative review, expert opinion, editorial, cadaveric studies, finite element analysis studies, or studies involving instability concurrent with ankle fractures were excluded as well as studies written in a language other than English. Only the risk factors presenting significant results in the studies were collected. The level of evidence for each article was classified according to Marx and colleagues[38,39] and the grade of evidence for each risk factor was assessed according to Wright and colleagues.[40] The risk factors were classified into mechanical, functional, personal, and environmental factors.

Following this process, 324 study titles were reviewed and 53 studies were selected. These 53 studies reported 68 significant findings for CAI risk factors, some of which were recurrently present in these studies (**Fig. 1**). The studies selected and grades of evidence for each risk factor are summarized in **Table 1**.

One of the most frequently reported risk factors was a prior history of ankle sprain and its severity.[41] Nevertheless, this factor is already in the mind of all providers and researchers and was not included as an independent risk factor because we consider it more of a consequence of CAI than a risk factor. The indirect consequences of this trauma will in any case be included in the risk factors (ie, rupture of the anterior talofibular ligament).

Foremost among several mechanical risk factors identified in the literature was ligamentous laxity. Involvement of the anterior talofibular and calcaneofibular ligaments, and associated laxities are commonly a focus in ankle sprain literature.[42–49] These two were indeed the most studied presenting, respectively, good and fair grades of evidence, but syndesmotic and subtalar laxity were also reported as CAI risk factors, although both of these were present with lower levels of evidence.[42,50,51] The presence of deltoid laxity as a risk factor for lateral instability is controversial. The latter is more frequently related to medial insufficiency associated with flatfoot or Progressive Collapsing Foot Deformity.[52] Its presence in lateral ankle instability may be biased by its strong pathomechanical connection with syndesmotic lesions.[53] It is more likely that syndesmotic laxity is the true risk factor for CAI and that deltoid insufficiency is indirectly related to CAI as it correlates with syndesmotic lesions.

The presence of decreased ankle dorsiflexion has also been recognized as a risk factor for CAI with fair evidence.[49,54–56] Our review does not specify whether this lack of dorsiflexion comes from an isolated gastrocnemius tightness, from a global retraction of the triceps surae, or from an anterior tibiotalar impingement.[57] Others were present with inferior evidences such as ankle and hindfoot varus or dysplasia involving the surrounding bones.[58–66] An anterior position of the fibula with respect to the tibia was also found as risk factor but we are unable to inform whether this is a consequence of ligamentous laxity or a real independent factor.[67,68]

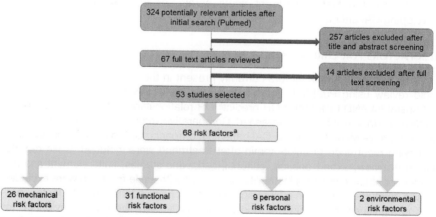

Fig. 1. Flow chart for structured literature review of CAI. [a]Some of them were present multiples times in different studies.

Table 1
Literature survey for risk factors of chronic ankle instability

Risk Factors	References	Level of Evidence	Grade of Evidence	Correctable?
Mechanical				
ATFL rupture—anterior drawer laxity	42–47	1 to 4	A—good	Yes
CFL rupture—varus tilt laxity	42–45,48,49	2 to 4	B—fair	Yes
Decreased ankle dorsiflexion	49,54–56	2 to 3	B—fair	Yes
Ankle and hindfoot varus	26,58–61	3 to 4	C—poor quality	Yes
Bony dysplasia (syndesmosis, talus, calcaneus)	62–66	3	C—poor quality	No
Anterior position of the fibula	Weerasekar et al.[67] 2021, Hubbard[68] 2006	3	C—poor quality	No
Syndesmotic and deltoid ligament laxity	Kim et al.[50] 2005	3	C—poor quality	Yes
Subtalar laxity (interosseous and cervical ligaments)	Denegar[42] 2002, Song et al.[51] 2021	4	I—insufficient	Yes
Functional				
Impaired neuromuscular control (including proprioception and balance deficits)	22,46,49,50,69–85	1 to 4	A—good	Yes
Altered gait patterns (walking, running, jumping…)	52,70,86–88	1 to 3	A—good	Yes
Strength deficit (evertors and plantarflexors)	22,46,47,89,90	1 to 4	A—good	Yes
Personal				
Increased BMI	46,47,70	1 to 3	A—good	Yes
Generalized laxity	91,92,104	1 to 3	A—good	No
Young age	Pourkazemi et al.[46] 2018, Fousekis[47] 2012	1	A—good	No
Kinesiophobia	Alshahrani[95] 2022	4	I—insufficient	Yes
Environmental				
Sport	Pourgharib Shahi et al.[93] 2021, Mailuhu et al.[94] 2019	2 to 3	B—fair	Yes

Abbreviations: ATFL, anterior talofibular ligament; BMI, body mass index; CFL, calcaneofibular ligament.

We divided the functional CAI risk factors into three groups according to the description by Donovan and Hertel[31,36]: impaired neuromuscular control, altered gait patterns, and strength deficit. Our results were consistent with those of these previous authors. Impaired neuromuscular control included notably proprioception, balance deficits, and delayed peroneal reaction time,[22,46,49,54,69-85] whereas altered gait patterns were a functional impairment when walking, running, or jumping.[52,73,86-88] Strength deficits were primarily represented by evertor weakness and less frequently by plantarflexor weakness.[22,46,47,89,90] These 3 groups of functional factors were all established with good evidence in the literature.

Personal and environmental factors were less studied, but good evidence was present regarding increased body mass index, generalized laxity, young age, and sports participation as risk factors for CAI,[46,47,70,91-94] whereas kinesiophobia was present with a low level of evidence.[95] It can also be noted that 75% of these risk factors can be medically or surgically corrected. Our opinion is that the management of CAI or acute sprains or prevention strategies must involve all these risk factors. As most of them can be present even before the first ankle sprain, we propose a model considering these risk factors as constitutional or consequential. Their detection and correction should be done either in anticipation before the initial injury or after the initial injury to allow the patient to cope with these factors and return to a normal life or as a treatment of CAI (**Fig. 2**).

In conclusion, functional risk factors are more studied and more validated than mechanical factors in the literature, but both should be included in the CAI management. We propose a model encompassing the mechanical and functional risk factors by considering them either as constitutional (present on the subject before the initial sprain) or consequential (developed after the trauma) with a cumulative effect of these risk factors. This model, unlike previous models, allows prevention and prophylactic management of constitutional risk factors to prevent initial ankle sprain, which could be effective for example in the sports field. We exposed an example of subject interaction with our cumulative risk factor model in **Fig. 2**.

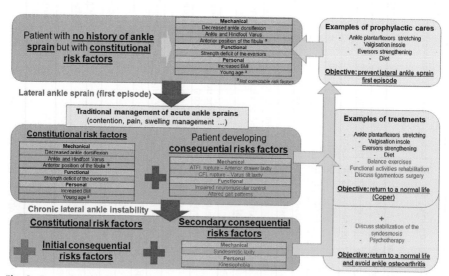

Fig. 2. Example of subject interaction with our cumulative risk factors model.

DIAGNOSING AND MEASURING CHRONIC ANKLE INSTABILITY

Diagnosing and measuring CAI is currently challenging. The most commonly used tools for this purpose are questionnaires like the Cumberland Ankle Instability Tool, the IdFAI, or the Foot and Ankle Ability Measure.[96,97] These questionnaires are limited by taking into account the history of ankle sprain in their items and therefore cannot be used in prevention. They are nonetheless routinely used in research to define study groups. The International Ankle Consortium has made recommendations on the selection criteria for patients with CAI including these questionnaires and their appropriate thresholds.[98]

As mentioned earlier, many studies focus only on the CAI mechanical or functional aspect. It is difficult to construct a study encompassing these two aspects as well as the personal and environmental risk factors that we have previously defined. In this way, sprain simulators have shown promising results.[99,100] These tools focus directly on the behavior of the ankle in the event of a sudden inversion motion. Assessment criteria typically used with these tools are maximum ankle inversion and maximum inversion velocity during the simulated trauma.[101–103] Ankle sprain simulators enable research encompassing the mechanical, functional, and all other CAI aspects. It can be discussed a theoretical risk of spraining the ankle during the simulated trauma, but according to Chu and colleagues[101] real ankle sprains involve inversion velocities over 500°/s and the use of a device simulating inversion trauma involving velocities less than 300°/s will exclude any risk of injury. A limitation of these studies is that most of them were performed in static positions or when landing, but not when walking and running, which might better reflect the actual conditions whereby ankle sprains occur.[99] These simulators could play a role in quantifying CAI as well as understanding the relative importance of each of its risk factors.

SUMMARY

CAI remains common and presents a significant socioeconomic burden. Progress in this area has been limited by the fact that different groups work on different CAI aspects (mainly mechanical and functional), whereas these factors fundamentally interact and need to be considered together. We performed a systematic review to collect the different risk factors for CAI and divided them into mechanical, functional, personal, and environmental for clarity, but all must be studied together. We have proposed a cumulative model including these risk factors that influence ankle sprains and CAI occurrences. Unlike previous CAI models, our model allows prophylactic management of patients at risk of ankle sprain, as well as CAI management. This model can be used for further research.

CLINICS CARE POINTS

- Alert patients with an ankle sprain sufficiently severe that they have sought medical care to concerns related to the risk for chronic ankle stability (CAI).
- Consider the multitude of risk factors for CAI when counseling patients who have suffered an ankle sprain.
- When evaluating CAI, consider both mechanical instability and functional impairment.
- Use established questionnaires to best capture functional impairment related to CAI.
- A course of physical therapy is warranted to address neuromuscular dysfunction for patients with CAI.

> • Mechanical risk factors, such as hindfoot varus or lack of ankle dorsiflexion, should be part of CAI management and can be corrected prophylactically.

DISCLOSURE

The authors have nothing relevant to disclose.

REFERENCES

1. Gribble PA, Bleakley CM, Caulfield BM, et al. Evidence review for the 2016 International Ankle Consortium consensus statement on the prevalence, impact and long-term consequences of lateral ankle sprains. Br J Sports Med 2016; 50(24):1496–505.
2. Herzog MM, Kerr ZY, Marshall SW, et al. Epidemiology of ankle sprains and chronic ankle instability. J Athletic Train 2019;54(6):603–10.
3. Lassiter TE, Malone TR, Garrett WE. Injury to the lateral ligaments of the ankle. Orthop Clin North Am 1989;20(4):629–40.
4. Wikstrom EA, Hubbard-Turner T, McKeon PO. Understanding and treating lateral ankle sprains and their consequences: a constraints-based approach. Sports Med 2013;43(6):385–93.
5. Wenning M, Gehring D, Mauch M, et al. Functional deficits in chronic mechanical ankle instability. J Orthop Surg Res 2020;15(1):304.
6. Spennacchio P, Meyer C, Karlsson J, et al. Evaluation modalities for the anatomical repair of chronic ankle instability. Knee Surg Sports Traumatol Arthrosc 2020;28(1):163–76.
7. Feger MA, Donovan L, Hart JM, et al. Lower extremity muscle activation in patients with or without chronic ankle instability during walking. J Athl Train 2015; 50(4):350–7.
8. Hubbard TJ, Kramer LC, Denegar CR, et al. Correlations among multiple measures of functional and mechanical instability in subjects with chronic ankle instability. J Athl Train 2007;42(3):361–6.
9. Houston MN, Hoch JM, Hoch MC. Patient-reported outcome measures in individuals with chronic ankle instability: a systematic review. J Athl Train 2015; 50(10):1019–33.
10. Lin CI, Houtenbos S, Lu YH, et al. The epidemiology of chronic ankle instability with perceived ankle instability- a systematic review. J Foot Ankle Res 2021;14(1):41.
11. Donovan L, Hetzel S, Laufenberg CR, et al. Prevalence and Impact of Chronic Ankle Instability in Adolescent Athletes. Orthopaedic J Sports Med 2020;8(2). https://doi.org/10.1177/2325967119900962. 232596711990096.
12. Hubbard-Turner T. Lack of medical treatment from a medical professional after an ankle sprain. J Athl Train 2019;54(6):671–5.
13. Michels F, Wastyn H, Pottel H, et al. The presence of persistent symptoms 12 months following a first lateral ankle sprain: a systematic review and meta-analysis. Foot Ankle Surg 2021. https://doi.org/10.1016/j.fas.2021.12.002. S1268-7731(21)00242-3.
14. Verhagen RA, de Keizer G, van Dijk CN. Long-term follow-up of inversion trauma of the ankle. Arch Orthop Trauma Surg 1995;114(2):92–6.
15. Taga I, Shino K, Inoue M, et al. Articular cartilage lesions in ankles with lateral ligament injury. An arthroscopic study. Am J Sports Med 1993;21(1):120–6 [discussion; 126-127].

16. Wang DY, Jiao C, Ao YF, et al. Risk factors for osteochondral lesions and osteo-phytes in chronic lateral ankle instability: a case series of 1169 patients. Orthop J Sports Med 2020;8(5). https://doi.org/10.1177/2325967120922821. 23259671 20922821.

17. Sugimoto K, Takakura Y, Okahashi K, et al. Chondral injuries of the ankle with recurrent lateral instability: an arthroscopic study. J Bone Joint Surg Am 2009; 91(1):99–106.

18. Valderrabano V, Hintermann B, Horisberger M, et al. Ligamentous posttraumatic ankle osteoarthritis. Am J Sports Med 2006;34(4):612–20.

19. Tropp H, Odenrick P, Gillquist J. Stabilometry recordings in functional and me-chanical instability of the ankle joint. Int J Sports Med 1985;6(3):180–2.

20. Wenning M, Schmal H. Chronic ankle instability - mechanical vs. Functional. Z Orthop Unfall 2022. https://doi.org/10.1055/a-1696-2503.

21. Brown CN, Rosen AB, Ko J. Ankle ligament laxity and stiffness in chronic ankle instability. Foot Ankle Int 2015;36(5):565–72.

22. Thompson C, Schabrun S, Romero R, et al. Factors contributing to chronic ankle instability: a systematic review and meta-analysis of systematic reviews. Sports Med 2018;48(1):189–205.

23. Tropp H. Commentary: functional ankle instability revisited. J Athl Train 2002; 37(4):512–5.

24. Freeman MA. Instability of the foot after injuries to the lateral ligament of the ankle. J Bone Joint Surg Br 1965;47(4):669–77.

25. Freeman MA, Dean MR, Hanham IW. The etiology and prevention of functional instability of the foot. J Bone Joint Surg Br 1965;47(4):678–85.

26. Yoshimoto K, Noguchi M, Maruki H, et al. Varus-Tilted Distal Tibial Plafond Is a Risk Factor for Recurrent Ankle Instability After Arthroscopic Lateral Ankle Lig-ament Repair. Foot Ankle Int 2022. https://doi.org/10.1177/10711007221077 099. 10711007221077100.

27. Ziai P, Benca E, Skrbensky GV, et al. The role of the medial ligaments in lateral stabilization of the ankle joint: an in vitro study. Knee Surg Sports Traumatol Ar-throsc 2015;23(7):1900–6.

28. Terada M, Pietrosimone BG, Gribble PA. Therapeutic interventions for increasing ankle dorsiflexion after ankle sprain: a systematic review. J Athl Train 2013;48(5): 696–709.

29. Hertel J. Functional instability following lateral ankle sprain. Sports Med 2000; 29(5):361–71.

30. Forestier N, Terrier R. Peroneal reaction time measurement in unipodal stance for two different destabilization axes. Clin Biomech 2011;26(7):766–71.

31. Hertel J, Corbett RO. An updated model of chronic ankle instability. J Athletic Train 2019;54(6):572–88.

32. Yoon DY, Moon SG, Jung HG, et al. Differences between subtalar instability and lateral ankle instability focusing on subtalar ligaments based on three dimen-sional isotropic magnetic resonance imaging. J Comput Assist Tomogr 2018; 42(4):566–73.

33. Wikstrom EA, Brown CN. Minimum reporting standards for copers in chronic ankle instability research. Sports Med 2014;44(2):251–68.

34. Doherty C, Bleakley C, Hertel J, et al. Dynamic balance deficits in individuals with chronic ankle instability compared with ankle sprain copers 1 year after a first-time lateral ankle sprain injury. Knee Surg Sports Traumatol Arthrosc 2016;24(4):1086–95.

35. Yu P, Mei Q, Xiang L, et al. Differences in the locomotion biomechanics and dynamic postural control between individuals with chronic ankle instability and copers: a systematic review. Sports Biomech 2022;21(4):531–49.

36. Donovan L, Hertel J. A new paradigm for rehabilitation of patients with chronic ankle instability. The Physician and Sportsmedicine 2012;40(4):41–51.

37. Miklovic TM, Donovan L, Protzuk OA, et al. Acute lateral ankle sprain to chronic ankle instability: a pathway of dysfunction. The Physician and Sportsmedicine 2018;46(1):116–22.

38. Marx RG, Wilson SM, Swiontkowski MF. Updating the Assignment of Levels of Evidence. The J Bone Joint Surg 2015;97(1):1–2.

39. Wright JG, Swiontkowski MF, Heckman JD. Introducing levels of evidence to the journal. J Bone Joint Surg Am 2003;85(1):1–3.

40. Wright JG, Einhorn TA, Heckman JD. Grades of recommendation. The J Bone Joint Surg 2005;87(9):1909–10.

41. Pourkazemi F, Hiller CE, Raymond J, et al. Predictors of chronic ankle instability after an index lateral ankle sprain: a systematic review. J Sci Med Sport 2014; 17(6):568–73.

42. Denegar CR, Hertel J, Fonseca J. The effect of lateral ankle sprain on dorsiflexion range of motion, posterior talar glide, and joint laxity. J Orthop Sports Phys Ther 2002;32(4):166–73.

43. Yamaguchi S, Akagi R, Kimura S, et al. Avulsion fracture of the distal fibula is associated with recurrent sprain after ankle sprain in children. Knee Surg Sports Traumatol Arthrosc 2019;27(9):2774–80.

44. Jung HG, Kim NR, Kim TH, et al. Magnetic resonance imaging and stress radiography in chronic lateral ankle instability. Foot Ankle Int 2017;38(6):621–6.

45. Halabchi F, Angoorani H, Mirshahi M, et al. The prevalence of selected intrinsic risk factors for ankle sprain among elite football and basketball players. Asian J Sports Med 2016;7(3). https://doi.org/10.5812/asjsm.35287.

46. Pourkazemi F, Hiller CE, Raymond J, et al. Predictors of recurrent sprains after an index lateral ankle sprain: a longitudinal study. Physiotherapy 2018;104(4): 430–7.

47. Fousekis K, Tsepis E, Vagenas G. Intrinsic risk factors of noncontact ankle sprains in soccer: a prospective study on 100 professional players. Am J Sports Med 2012;40(8):1842–50.

48. Pacheco J, Guerra-Pinto F, Araújo L, et al. Chronic ankle instability has no correlation with the number of ruptured ligaments in severe anterolateral sprain: a systematic review and meta-analysis. Knee Surg Sports Traumatol Arthrosc 2021;29(11):3512–24.

49. Rosen A, Ko J, Brown C. A multivariate assessment of clinical contributions to the severity of perceived dysfunction measured by the cumberland ankle instability tool. Int J Sports Med 2016;37(14):1154–8.

50. Kim JS, Young KW, Cho HK, et al. Concomitant syndesmotic instability and medial ankle instability are risk factors for unsatisfactory outcomes in patients with chronic ankle instability. Arthroscopy 2015;31(8):1548–56.

51. Song WT, Lee J, Lee JH, et al. A high rate of talocalcaneal interosseous ligament tears was found in chronic lateral ankle instability with sinus tarsi pain. Knee Surg Sports Traumatol Arthrosc 2021;29(11):3543–50.

52. Myerson MS, Thordarson DB, Johnson JE, et al. Classification and nomenclature: progressive collapsing foot deformity. Foot Ankle Int 2020;41(10):1271–6.

53. Spennacchio P, Seil R, Gathen M, et al. Diagnosing instability of ligamentous syndesmotic injuries: A biomechanical perspective. Clin Biomech (Bristol, Avon) 2021;84:105312.

54. Bączkowicz D, Falkowski K, Majorczyk E. Assessment of relationships between joint motion quality and postural control in patients with chronic ankle joint instability. J Orthop Sports Phys Ther 2017;47(8):570–7.

55. Grindstaff TL, Dolan N, Morton SK. Ankle dorsiflexion range of motion influences Lateral Step Down Test scores in individuals with chronic ankle instability. Phys Ther Sport 2017;23:75–81.

56. De Ridder R, Willems T, Vanrenterghem J, et al. Multi-segment foot landing kinematics in subjects with chronic ankle instability. Clin Biomech (Bristol, Avon) 2015;30(6):585–92.

57. DiGiovanni CW, Kuo R, Tejwani N, et al. Isolated gastrocnemius tightness. J Bone Joint Surg Am 2002;84(6):962–70.

58. Sugimoto K, Samoto N, Takakura Y, et al. Varus tilt of the tibial plafond as a factor in chronic ligament instability of the ankle. Foot Ankle Int 1997;18(7):402–5.

59. Shim DW, Suh JW, Park KH, et al. Diagnosis and operation results for chronic lateral ankle instability with subtle cavovarus deformity and a peek-a-boo heel sign. Yonsei Med J 2020;61(7):635–9.

60. Lintz F, Bernasconi A, Baschet L, et al. Relationship between chronic lateral ankle instability and hindfoot varus using weight-bearing cone beam computed tomography. Foot Ankle Int 2019;40(10):1175–81.

61. Van Bergeyk AB, Younger A, Carson B. CT analysis of hindfoot alignment in chronic lateral ankle instability. Foot Ankle Int 2002;23(1):37–42.

62. Ataoğlu MB, Tokgöz MA, Köktürk A, et al. Radiologic evaluation of the effect of distal tibiofibular joint anatomy on arthroscopically proven ankle instability. Foot Ankle Int 2020;41(2):223–8.

63. Tümer N, Vuurberg G, Blankevoort L, et al. Typical shape differences in the subtalar joint bones between subjects with chronic ankle instability and controls. J Orthop Res 2019;37(9):1892–902.

64. Magerkurth O, Frigg A, Hintermann B, et al. Frontal and lateral characteristics of the osseous configuration in chronic ankle instability. Br J Sports Med 2010; 44(8):568–72.

65. Frigg A, Frigg R, Hintermann B, et al. The biomechanical influence of tibio-talar containment on stability of the ankle joint. Knee Surg Sports Traumatol Arthr 2007;15(11):1355–62.

66. Frigg A, Magerkurth O, Valderrabano V, et al. The effect of osseous ankle configuration on chronic ankle instability. Br J Sports Med 2007;41(7):420–4.

67. Weerasekara I, Osmotherly PG, Snodgrass S, et al. Is the fibula positioned anteriorly in weight-bearing in individuals with chronic ankle instability? A case control study. J Man Manip Ther 2021;29(3):168–75.

68. Hubbard TJ, Hertel J, Sherbondy P. Fibular position in individuals with self-reported chronic ankle instability. J Orthop Sports Phys Ther 2006;36(1):3–9.

69. Yoshida T, Suzuki T. Relationship between chronic ankle sprain instability and ultrasonographic evaluation of the peroneus during a single-leg standing task. J Phys Ther Sci 2020;32(1):33–7.

70. Vuurberg G, Altink N, Rajai M, et al. Weight, BMI and stability are risk factors associated with lateral ankle sprains and chronic ankle instability: a meta-analysis. J ISAKOS 2019;4(6):313–27.

71. Thompson CS, Hiller CE, Schabrun SM. Altered spinal-level sensorimotor control related to pain and perceived instability in people with chronic ankle instability. J Sci Med Sport 2019;22(4):425–9.

72. Silva DCF, Macedo R, Montes AM, et al. Does the cleat model interfere with ankle sprain risk factors in artificial grass? Clin Biomech (Bristol, Avon) 2019; 63:119–26.

73. Ko J, Rosen AB, Brown CN. Functional performance tests identify lateral ankle sprain risk: a prospective pilot study in adolescent soccer players. Scand J Med Sci Sports 2018;28(12):2611–6.

74. Sierra-Guzmán R, Jiménez F, Abián-Vicén J. Predictors of chronic ankle instability: analysis of peroneal reaction time, dynamic balance and isokinetic strength. Clin Biomech (Bristol, Avon) 2018;54:28–33.

75. Mineta S, Inami T, Mariano R, et al. High lateral plantar pressure is related to an increased tibialis anterior/fibularis longus activity ratio in patients with recurrent lateral ankle sprain. Open Access J Sports Med 2017;8:123–31.

76. Doherty C, Bleakley C, Hertel J, et al. Recovery from a first-time lateral ankle sprain and the predictors of chronic ankle instability: a prospective cohort analysis. Am J Sports Med 2016;44(4):995–1003.

77. Pourkazemi F, Hiller C, Raymond J, et al. Using balance tests to discriminate between participants with a recent index lateral ankle sprain and healthy control participants: a cross-sectional study. J Athl Train 2016;51(3):213–22.

78. Powell MR, Powden CJ, Houston MN, et al. Plantar cutaneous sensitivity and balance in individuals with and without chronic ankle instability. Clin J Sport Med 2014;24(6):490–6.

79. de Noronha M, França LC, Haupenthal A, et al. Intrinsic predictive factors for ankle sprain in active university students: a prospective study. Scand J Med Sci Sports 2013;23(5):541–7.

80. Suda EY, Sacco IC. Altered leg muscle activity in volleyball players with functional ankle instability during a sideward lateral cutting movement. Phys Ther Sport 2011;12(4):164–70.

81. Sefton JM, Hicks-Little CA, Hubbard TJ, et al. Sensorimotor function as a predictor of chronic ankle instability. Clin Biomech (Bristol, Avon) 2009;24(5):451–8.

82. Palmieri-Smith RM, Hopkins JT, Brown TN. Peroneal activation deficits in persons with functional ankle instability. Am J Sports Med 2009;37(5):982–8.

83. Mitchell A, Dyson R, Hale T, et al. Biomechanics of ankle instability. Part 2: postural sway-reaction time relationship. Med Sci Sports Exerc 2008;40(8): 1522–8.

84. Konradsen L. Factors contributing to chronic ankle instability: kinesthesia and joint position sense. J Athl Train 2002;37(4):381–5.

85. Lentell G, Katzman LL, Walters MR. The relationship between muscle function and ankle stability. J Orthop Sports Phys Ther 1990;11(12):605–11.

86. Lee I, Lee SY, Ha S. Alterations of lower extremity function, health-related quality of life, and spatiotemporal gait parameters among individuals with chronic ankle instability. Phys Ther Sport 2021;51:22–8.

87. Ko J, Rosen AB, Brown CN. Functional performance deficits in adolescent athletes with a history of lateral ankle sprain(s). Phys Ther Sport 2018;33:125–32.

88. Liu K, Dierkes C, Blair L. A new jump-landing protocol identifies differences in healthy, coper, and unstable ankles in collegiate athletes. Sports Biomech 2016;15(3):245–54.

89. Hou ZC, Miao X, Ao YF, et al. Characteristics and predictors of muscle strength deficit in mechanical ankle instability. BMC Musculoskelet Disord 2020; 21(1):730.
90. Docherty CL, Arnold BL, Hurwitz S. Contralateral force sense deficits are related to the presence of functional ankle instability. J Orthop Res 2006;24(7):1412–9.
91. Xu HX, Lee KB. Modified broström procedure for chronic lateral ankle instability in patients with generalized joint laxity. Am J Sports Med 2016;44(12):3152–7.
92. Park KH, Lee JW, Suh JW, et al. Generalized ligamentous laxity is an independent predictor of poor outcomes after the modified broström procedure for chronic lateral ankle instability. Am J Sports Med 2016;44(11):2975–83.
93. Pourgharib Shahi MH, Selk Ghaffari M, Mansournia MA, et al. Risk factors influencing the incidence of ankle sprain among elite football and basketball players: a prospective study. Foot Ankle Spec 2021;14(6):482–8.
94. Mailuhu AKE, Oei EHG, van Ochten JM, et al. Subgroup characteristics of patients with chronic ankle instability in primary care. J Sci Med Sport 2019; 22(8):866–70.
95. Alshahrani MS, Reddy RS. Relationship between kinesiophobia and ankle joint position sense and postural control in individuals with chronic ankle instability-A cross-sectional study. Int J Environ Res Public Health 2022;19(5):2792.
96. Hiller CE, Refshauge KM, Bundy AC, et al. The cumberland ankle instability tool: a report of validity and reliability testing. Arch Phys Med Rehabil 2006;87(9): 1235–41.
97. Simon J, Donahue M, Docherty C. Development of the identification of functional ankle instability (IdFAI). Foot Ankle Int 2012;33(9):755–63.
98. Gribble PA, Delahunt E, Bleakley CM, et al. Selection criteria for patients with chronic ankle instability in controlled research: a position statement of the international ankle consortium. J Athl Train 2014;49(1):121–7.
99. Ha SCW, Fong DTP, Chan KM. Review of ankle inversion sprain simulators in the biomechanics laboratory. Asia-Pacific J Sports Med Arthrosc Rehabil Technology 2015;2(4):114–21.
100. Chan YY, Fong DTP, Yung PSH, et al. A mechanical supination sprain simulator for studying ankle supination sprain kinematics. J Biomech 2008;41(11):2571–4.
101. Chu VWS, Fong DTP, Chan YY, et al. Differentiation of ankle sprain motion and common sporting motion by ankle inversion velocity. J Biomech 2010;43(10): 2035–8.
102. Simpson JD, Stewart EM, Mosby AM, et al. Lower-extremity kinematics during ankle inversion perturbations: a novel experimental protocol that simulates an unexpected lateral ankle sprain mechanism. J Sport Rehabil 2019;28(6): 593–600.
103. Simpson JD, Stewart EM, Turner AJ, et al. Neuromuscular control in individuals with chronic ankle instability: a comparison of unexpected and expected ankle inversion perturbations during a single leg drop-landing. Hum Movement Sci 2019;64:133–41.
104. Saki F, Yalfani A, Fousekis K, et al. Anatomical risk factors of lateral ankle sprain in adolescent athletes: A prospective cohort study. Phys Ther Sport 2021;48: 26–34.

Effect of Braces on Performance in the Context of Chronic Ankle Instability

Claire E. Hiller, PhD, MAppSc, BAppSc*, Paula R. Beckenkamp, PhD

KEYWORDS

- Chronic ankle instability • Ankle brace • External ankle support
- Functional performance • Balance

KEY POINTS

- Braces are effective to prevent recurrent ankle sprains.
- Braces do not impede functional performance and at times enhance performance in people with chronic ankle instability.
- Hopping, jumping, and dynamic balance activities are most likely to be improved.
- Clinicians should have a range of ankle braces to recommend, to accommodate patient preference and comfort, and so ensure compliance.

INTRODUCTION

Ankle sprains are prevalent, particularly for people involved in indoor and court sports, with lateral ankle sprain being the most common type of sprain.[1] It has been reported that about 40% of people who had a significant first-time ankle sprain develop ongoing symptoms, known as chronic ankle instability (CAI), for more than 1 year after injury.[2] External ankle supports, in the form of ankle braces or tape, are recommended for both primary and secondary prevention of ankle sprains to provide protection following an acute ankle sprain[3] or surgery for CAI[4] and during return to normal or sporting activity.[3] However, the use of ankle external support, such as an ankle brace, should not be the only intervention selected to target balance and postural stability in people with CAI.[3] This article discusses the use of external ankle braces, specifically semirigid, soft-shell, or lace-up ankle braces, in people with CAI and the effects, or not, of wearing a brace on functional performance.

DEFINITION OF CHRONIC ANKLE INSTABILITY

CAI is the term used to refer to a combination of persistent symptoms that are commonly seen in people after they have experienced an ankle sprain. CAI commonly

Sydney School of Health Sciences, The University of Sydney, D18 Susan Wakil Health Building, Western Avenue, Camperdown NSW 2006, Sydney, Australia
* Corresponding author.
E-mail address: claire.hiller@sydney.edu.au

Foot Ankle Clin N Am 28 (2023) 145–154
https://doi.org/10.1016/j.fcl.2022.10.006
foot.theclinics.com

includes episodes and/or the subjective feeling of ankle join instability (also reported as the feeling of the ankle "giving way"), and/or recurrent sprains, observed for longer than 1 year following the initial sprain.[5] Other ongoing problems associated with CAI include pain, functional impairments, and reduced physical activity participation.[6]

CHRONIC ANKLE INSTABILITY IMPAIRMENTS

Many studies have reported associated impairments that have been found in people with CAI.[7–9] More recently, the CAI model has been updated[10] and includes a variety of impairments such as joint-related impairments (mechanical instability, restricted range of motion, particularly of dorsiflexion range, and reduced accessory movements of the ankle), reduced proprioception and balance, pain, subjective feeling of instability, reduced self-reported function, and personal and environmental factors, such as age and health care access, respectively. The investigators highlighted that, although these are common impairments observed in people with CAI, they are not all necessarily present in everyone that presents with CAI.[10]

The impact of CAI can be seen in many aspects of someone's health. It has been established that CAI negatively affects quality of life and function and the ability to fully engage in physical activity.[11–13] A previous study[13] demonstrated that people with CAI engaged in less moderate-to-vigorous physical activity per week when compared with people without a history of ankle sprains (94.2 ± 28.6 vs 212.5 ± 38.5 minutes per week) measured by the short form of the International Physical Activity Questionnaire, and reduced step count as measured by a pedometer (6694.5 ± 1603.4 vs 8831.0 ± 1290.0 steps per day).[13]

It has been demonstrated that people with CAI are also more prone to develop post-traumatic ankle osteoarthritis, with studies reporting early signs of joint degeneration and chondral lesions in people with CAI.[14,15] Research has also demonstrated that people with end-stage post-traumatic ankle osteoarthritis are usually younger, and the progression of the condition tends to be faster when compared with other joints, such as knee and hip osteoarthritis.[16]

WHY BRACE?

Several recommendations have been made over the years on the use of ankle braces; however, many clinical practice guidelines and consensus statements that include advice on the use of brace are primarily directed to ankle sprains[17–19] rather than to CAI.[3,4,20] Ankle braces are used in people with CAI to address various impairments and, thus, to prevent reinjury, support the ankle during functional performance and in rehabilitation protocols after surgery.

Braces have been recommended for both primary and secondary prevention of ankle sprains (Level 1 evidence, highest level).[3] A systematic review of randomized controlled trials examining the use of a brace compared with a no brace condition in athletic ankle reinjury, demonstrated a risk ratio in favor of ankle brace use of 0.53 (95% confidence interval 0.32–0.88) for primary prevention, and 0.37 (0.24–0.58) for secondary prevention.[21] Although this outcome was ankle injury rather than sprain, most athletic ankle injuries are lateral ankle sprains.[1] If you consider studies only investigating repeated ankle sprains, then an overview of systematic reviews found there was unanimous consensus that braces prevented recurrent sprains.[22]

Braces are also used during rehabilitation protocols to provide support to the ankle during healing[23] and subsequently to provide support during physical activity and return to work. This support may be to restrict joint range of motion, protect joint integrity, provide proprioceptive feedback, or improve perceived ankle instability, and, thus, improve performance or increase physical activity participation, and not just to prevent an ankle sprain.

HOW DO BRACES WORK?

Ankle braces are suggested to act in several ways. Braces provide restriction to ankle joint range of motion, particularly by restricting excessive inversion range of the subtalar joint, in both uninjured people[24,25] and in people with CAI[24] or a history of ankle injuries.[26] The restrictions are more pronounced in people with CAI than in uninjured controls,[24] and it has been shown that although an ankle brace reduces ankle inversion range during a sudden ankle inversion, normal sagittal movement at the ankle and knee is maintained in people with a history of lateral ankle sprain.[27] Braces have also been shown to restrict excessive plantar flexion in the swing phase of walking in people with CAI.[28]

Ankle braces also act to protect ankle joint integrity.[29] In a study involving 25 participants with mechanical ankle instability, it was demonstrated that wearing an ankle brace improved joint congruency when measured by 3D stress MRI, thus reducing the talar load, a factor known to be involved in the development of osteochondral, and/or degenerative changes to the ankle joint.[29]

It has been hypothesized that prophylactic ankle stabilizers could act by enhancing proprioceptive awareness of the ankle in people with functional ankle instability.[30] Lace-up ankle braces improved neuromuscular control during agility tests (single-leg drop vertical jump, single-leg squat, and Y-excursion tests) in an active healthy population.[31] The investigators observed no difference in outcomes between the lace-up brace and a silicone ankle sleeve, which indicated that a possible proprioceptive effect was associated with wearing a brace.[31] Although it should be noted that a systematic review of the effect of braces on proprioception in people with CAI or a history of ankle sprain did not find that braces enhanced or diminished proprioception as measured by joint position sense or movement detection.[32]

Ankle braces have also been shown to work psychologically. Wearing a brace, as well as ankle tape, has enhanced a person's confidence, reassurance, and a sense of stability of the ankle during dynamic activities.[33]

PERFORMANCE EFFECTS OF BRACES

Barriers to brace use include the idea that the ankle brace will impede functional performance. Functional performance can be considered to include balance, jumping, hopping, running, agility, and sport-specific movements. Performance can be considered from the aspect of biomechanics and function. Most of the studies investigating the effect of braces on functional performance use an uninjured population. A systematic review of the effect of braces on dynamic balance found that braces had a weak negative or no effect in healthy participants.[34] Similarly, studies of static balance in healthy participants have found no[25,35,36] or a negative effect.[35] In a systematic review on the effects of ankle support on functional activities that did not include balance activities,[37] only 4 of 17 included studies investigated the effects in an ankle injured population. The main findings from meta-analyses in this systematic review were that a lace-up style brace impeded sprint and agility speed and lace-up and semirigid braces decreased vertical jump height. There was no separate examination of the ankle-injured population. Therefore, overall, braces may have no or a negative effect on function in healthy participants, but the effect of bracing on performance in participants with CAI may be variable to positive across these different categories.

Biomechanics

A recent systematic review investigated the effects of ankle supports on lower limb biomechanics during functional tasks, which included walking, running, jumping, cutting, or landing.[38] Meta-analyses found no effect of braces on peak vertical ground reaction force during landing from a jump, peak plantar flexion angle during stance in running, or peak medial or vertical ground reaction force or ankle inversion angle at contact in a cutting task (**Fig. 1**). No studies investigated biomechanics in the transverse plane, which is disappointing given that internal rotation has been identified as one common aspect in ankle sprain injury mechanism.[39,40]

From the 31 studies identified in the systematic review[38] that tested braces, only five explicitly included participants with CAI.[27,30,41–43] Of these, none found an effect of braces on the biomechanical variables investigated, including two that compared a group of people with CAI with control participants.[42,43] Given the limited biomechanical variables investigated, small sample sizes and different braces, no conclusions can currently be drawn about the effect of bracing on biomechanics during functional activities in people with CAI.

Function

Balance

Balance can be considered in terms of static and dynamic balance. Single-leg static balance has been shown not to be affected[44] or improved[45] in people with CAI when wearing lace-up or soft-shell braces. Dynamic balance, measured using the Star Excursion Balance test (SEBT) or Y test, has been shown to be improved with the application of braces in people with CAI.[34,46] A strong positive effect of bracing, using four different brace types, was noted in a recent systematic review, which pooled the SEBT direction results.[34] Interestingly, a network meta-analysis that only looked at the posteromedial direction of the SEBT found no effect.[46] As both reviews used data from the same two studies, it seems that braces may assist with some aspects of dynamic balance, but not others, in people with CAI.

Agility

Various agility measures have been investigated when considering the use of braces in participants with CAI. These include shuttle run,[47] a modified Japan test,[48] figure 8,[49,50] and sidesteps over 8 m.[51] None of these studies showed that wearing a brace (semirigid or soft-shell) altered the amount of time taken for participants with CAI to complete the tested course.

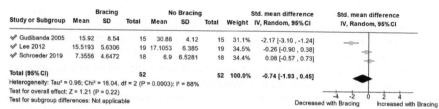

Fig. 1. Ankle inversion angle at initial contact or early stance during cutting movement: bracing versus control. (Tomas Megalaa, Claire E. Hiller, Giovanni E. Ferreira, Paula R. Beckenkamp, Evangelos Pappas, The effect of ankle supports on lower limb biomechanics during functional tasks: A systematic review with meta-analysis, Journal of Science and Medicine in Sport, 25 (7), 2022, 615-630, https://doi.org/10.1016/j.jsams.2022.02.008.[38]).

Hopping

Hopping has been investigated using a course with sloped surfaces, or hopping in various directions, and times have either improved or shown no change when a participant with CAI wore an ankle brace. Two studies investigated hopping around a tight course landing on surfaces inclined in four directions to ensure landing in plantar flexion, dorsiflexion, inversion, and eversion.[45,52] The earlier study found a significantly quicker time around the hopping course when wearing a lace-up or soft-shell brace,[45] however, the later study, with 10 more recent braces, did not find a difference, except for a rigid brace, which increased the hopping time.[52] A hopping study akin to more recent dance style mats where participants hopped from a central square to each of four outside squares in response to a lit signal, found that participants with CAI completed the random sequence quicker, and spent less time in contact with the squares when wearing a semirigid brace.[48]

Jumping

A vertical jump is the most commonly investigated jump in functional performance. Five studies have investigated the vertical jump in participants with CAI or history of ankle sprain, and all of them found no significant difference between wearing and not wearing a brace.[26,47,49,50,52] The only exception was Gunay and colleagues,[26] who found that, although a single-leg vertical jump did not show a difference, the double-leg vertical jump resulted in a higher jump in participants wearing an Aircast brace (style not reported) than when not wearing a brace. Although a broad jump has been investigated in uninjured participants, showing a decrease in performance[53] when wearing a lace-up brace, the effect does not seem to have been investigated in participants with CAI.

Sprint

Only Gross and colleagues[49] seem to have investigated the effects of a brace on sprint times in participants with CAI. They investigated the effect of wearing two different semirigid braces compared with no brace while completing a straight 40-m sprint and found no difference in sprint times between conditions. These results were similar to a previous study by the same investigators using the same braces in participants who had not had an injury in the previous 6 months.[54]

POSTSURGICAL EFFECTS OF BRACES

When CAI has failed conservative treatment, suggested to be 3 to 6 months of functional rehabilitation including bracing,[4,55] surgery may be indicated. The use of braces as part of postsurgical protocols has not been researched. Indeed, a couple of recent systematic reviews of postoperative protocols for CAI state that most protocols are of level 5 evidence.[56,57] Braces were minimally mentioned as being used in the post-immobilization phase[4,56,57] and so guidance during rehabilitation from use in conservative treatment of CAI should be used.

DISCUSSION

There is surprisingly little research undertaken on the effects of brace use in people with CAI, given that they would be expected to be the among the highest users of braces. The research that has been done spans a wide range of years and many different brace types and brands, making definitive conclusions difficult. However, no studies have found a deleterious effect on performance of wearing soft-shell, semirigid, or lace-up ankle braces in people with CAI, and some found improvements in performance. Improvements occurred in some dynamic balance, jumping, and hopping tasks. In the end, braces are effective for prevention of sprains, rehabilitation, and return to sport and physical activity[3,18] and should be recommended for people with CAI.

The best brace is the brace that people will wear. The most appropriate brace is selected based on findings from the history, physical examination, individual needs, and patients' preferences.[3] Patients' preferences can be influenced by several factors. Apart from perceptions that performance could be affected, there are perceptions that braces can cause injuries higher up the kinetic chain,[58] esthetics, appearance of weakness, and discomfort.[59] Not to mention the lack of awareness of the effectiveness of ankle braces. Unfortunately for clinicians, brace preference is also very individual.[60]

The idea that restricting ankle movement will lead to impacts and injury higher up the chain is plausible theoretically. One study of female basketball players wearing two different braces (lace-up and hinged) undertaking a cutting task[61] found that both braces increased knee internal rotation and abduction angles, which could lead to increased knee injuries. However, a study by McGuine et al.[62] investigating the use of a lace-up brace to prevent injuries in high school basketball players found a decrease in ankle sprains but no change to the rate of acute knee or other lower limb injuries. This is an area that warrants further investigation.

The few studies that have investigated personal preference in braces have found that many factors can be barriers. It is interesting that in one study of young basketball players, esthetics was the major consideration, followed by the appearance of weakness,[59] however, it is not known if this is true for older people. In another study of different athlete groups, the type of brace (compression, lace-up, semirigid) that was preferred varied by sporting group, along with the perceptions of stability and comfort.[60] It should be noted that clinicians also have concerns about recommending brace use, of which the main concern is ankle musculature weakness[63] and this factor had a significant correlation with not recommending a brace after an initial ankle sprain. This is despite a lack of evidence that brace use results in muscle weakness.

Clinicians should consider a range of braces to recommend depending on the goal of use, and providing for individual preference, secure in the knowledge that for people with CAI functional performance is unlikely to be affected, and, in fact, may be enhanced.

DISCLOSURE

Claire Hiller has received braces from KISS Pty Ltd for research studies. KISS had no input on the material in this article.

REFERENCES

1. Doherty C, Delahunt E, Caulfield B, et al. The incidence and prevalence of ankle sprain injury: a systematic review and meta-analysis of prospective epidemiological studies. Sports Med 2014;44(1):123–40.

2. Doherty C, Bleakley C, Hertel J, et al. Recovery from a first-time lateral ankle sprain and the predictors of chronic ankle instability: a prospective cohort analysis. Am J Sports Med 2016;44(4):995–1003.

3. Martin RL, Davenport TE, Fraser JJ, et al. Ankle stability and movement coordination impairments: lateral ankle ligament sprains revision 2021. J Orthop Sports Phys Ther 2021;51(4):1–80.

4. Song Y, Li H, Sun C, et al. Clinical guidelines for the surgical management of chronic lateral ankle instability: a consensus reached by systematic review of the available data. Orthop J Sports Med 2019;7(9). 2325967119873852.

5. Gribble PA, Delahunt E, Bleakley C, et al. Selection criteria for patients with chronic ankle instability in controlled research: a position statement of the International Ankle Consortium. Br J Sports Med 2014;48(13):1014–8.

6. Gribble PA, Bleakley CM, Caulfield BM, et al. Evidence review for the 2016 International Ankle Consortium consensus statement on the prevalence, impact and long-term consequences of lateral ankle sprains. Br J Sports Med 2016;50(24): 1496–505.

7. Freeman MA, Dean MR, Hanham IW. The etiology and prevention of functional instability of the foot. J Bone Joint Surg Br 1965;47(4):678–85.

8. Hertel J. Functional instability following lateral ankle sprain. Sports Med 2000; 29(5):361–71.

9. Hiller CE, Kilbreath SL, Refshauge KM. Chronic ankle instability: evolution of the model. J Athl Train 2011;46(2):133–41.

10. Hertel J, Corbett RO. An updated model of chronic ankle instability. J Athl Train 2019;54(6):572–88.

11. Houston MN, Hoch JM, Hoch MC. Patient-reported outcome measures in individuals with chronic ankle instability: a systematic review. J Athl Train 2015;50(10): 1019–33.

12. Houston MN, Van Lunen BL, Hoch MC. Health-related quality of life in individuals with chronic ankle instability. J Athl Train 2014;49(6):758–63.

13. Hubbard-Turner T, Turner MJ. Physical activity levels in college students with chronic ankle instability. J Athl Train 2015;50(7):742–7.

14. Golditz T, Steib S, Pfeifer K, et al. Functional ankle instability as a risk factor for osteoarthritis: using T2-mapping to analyze early cartilage degeneration in the ankle joint of young athletes. Osteoarthritis Cartilage 2014;22(10):1377–85.

15. Lee M, Kwon JW, Choi WJ, et al. Comparison of outcomes for osteochondral lesions of the talus with and without chronic lateral ankle instability. Foot Ankle Int 2015;36(9):1050–7.

16. Valderrabano V, Hintermann B, Horisberger M, et al. Ligamentous posttraumatic ankle osteoarthritis. Am J Sports Med 2006;34(4):612–20.

17. Kaminski TW, Hertel J, Amendola N, et al. National Athletic Trainers' Association position statement: conservative management and prevention of ankle sprains in athletes. J Athl Train 2013;48(4):528–45.

18. Richie DH, Izadi FE. Return to play after an ankle sprain: guidelines for the podiatric physician. Clin Podiatr Med Surg 2015;32(2):195–215.

19. Vuurberg G, Hoorntje A, Wink LM, et al. Diagnosis, treatment and prevention of ankle sprains: update of an evidence-based clinical guideline. Br J Sports Med 2018;52(15):956.

20. Czajka CM, Tran E, Cai AN, et al. Ankle sprains and instability. Med Clin North Am 2014;98(2):313–29.

21. Barelds I, van den Broek AG, Huisstede BMA. Ankle bracing is effective for primary and secondary prevention of acute ankle injuries in athletes: a systematic review and meta-analyses. Sports Med 2018;48(12):2775–84.

22. Doherty C, Bleakley C, Delahunt E, et al. Treatment and prevention of acute and recurrent ankle sprain: an overview of systematic reviews with meta-analysis. Br J Sports Med 2017;51(2):113–25.

23. Vuurberg G, Altink N, Rajai M, et al. Weight, BMI and stability are risk factors associated with lateral ankle sprains and chronic ankle instability: a meta-analysis. J ISAKOS 2019;4(6):313–27.

24. Fuerst P, Gollhofer A, Wenning M, et al. People with chronic ankle instability benefit from brace application in highly dynamic change of direction movements. J Foot Ankle Res 2021;14(1):13.

25. Parsley A, Chinn L, Lee SY, et al. Effect of 3 different ankle braces on functional performance and ankle range of motion. Athl Train Sports Health Care 2013;5(2):69–75.

26. Gunay S, Karaduman A, Ozturk BB. Effects of Aircast brace and elastic bandage on physical performance of athletes after ankle injuries. Acta Orthop Traumatol Turc 2014;48(1):10–6.

27. Agres AN, Chrysanthou M, Raffalt PC. The effect of ankle bracing on kinematics in simulated sprain and drop landings: a double-blind, placebo-controlled study. Am J Sports Med 2019;47(6):1480–7.

28. Migel K, Wikstrom E. Gait biomechanics following taping and bracing in patients with chronic ankle instability: a critically appraised topic. J Sport Rehabil 2020;29(3):373–6.

29. Eberbach H, Gehring D, Lange T, et al. Efficacy of a semirigid ankle brace in reducing mechanical ankle instability evaluated by 3D stress-MRI. J Orthop Surg Res 2021;16(1):620.

30. Wikstrom EA, Arrigenna MA, Tillman MD, et al. Dynamic postural stability in subjects with braced, functionally unstable ankles. J Athl Train 2006;41(3):245–50.

31. Cinque ME, Bodendorfer BM, Shu HT, et al. The effect of silicone ankle sleeves and lace-up ankle braces on neuromuscular control, joint torque, and cutting agility. J Orthop 2020;20:359–66.

32. Raymond J, Nicholson LL, Hiller CE, et al. The effect of ankle taping or bracing on proprioception in functional ankle instability: a systematic review and meta-analysis. J Sci Med Sport 2012;15(5):386–92.

33. Simon J, Donahue M. Effect of ankle taping or bracing on creating an increased sense of confidence, stability, and reassurance when performing a dynamic-balance task. J Sport Rehabil 2013;22(3):229–33.

34. Reyburn RJ, Powden CJ. Dynamic balance measures in healthy and chronic ankle instability participants while wearing ankle braces: systematic review with meta-analysis. J Sport Rehabil 2020;30(4):660–7.

35. Bennell KL, Goldie PA. The differential effects of external ankle support on postural control. J Orthop Sports Phys Ther 1994;20(6):287–95.

36. Maeda N, Urabe Y, Tsutsumi S, et al. Effect of Semi-Rigid and Soft Ankle braces on static and dynamic postural stability in young male adults. J Sports Sci Med 2016;15(2):352–7.

37. Cordova ML, Scott BD, Ingersoll CD, et al. Effects of ankle support on lower-extremity functional performance: a meta-analysis. Med Sci Sports Exerc 2005;37(4):635–41.

38. Megalaa T, Hiller CE, Ferreira GE, et al. The effect of ankle supports on lower limb biomechanics during functional tasks: a systematic review with meta-analysis. J Sci Med Sport 2022;25(7):615–30.

39. Fong DT, Ha SC, Mok KM, et al. Kinematics analysis of ankle inversion ligamentous sprain injuries in sports: five cases from televised tennis competitions. Am J Sports Med 2012;40(11):2627–32.

40. Panagiotakis E, Mok KM, Fong DT, et al. Biomechanical analysis of ankle ligamentous sprain injury cases from televised basketball games: understanding

when, how and why ligament failure occurs. J Sci Med Sport 2017;20(12): 1057–61.

41. Donovan L, Hart JM, Saliba S, et al. Effects of ankle destabilization devices and rehabilitation on gait biomechanics in chronic ankle instability patients: a randomized controlled trial. Phys Ther Sport 2016;21:46–56.

42. Spaulding SJ, Livingston LA, Hartsell HD. The influence of external orthotic support on the adaptive gait characteristics of individuals with chronically unstable ankles. Gait Posture 2003;17(2):152–8.

43. Zhang S, Wortley M, Silvernail JF, et al. Do ankle braces provide similar effects on ankle biomechanical variables in subjects with and without chronic ankle instability during landing? J Sport Health Sci 2012;1(2):114–20.

44. Wu J, Lu A. Effects of different types of ankle brace on the static postural stability in patients with functional ankle instability. Chin J Sports Med 2017;6:232–5.

45. Jerosch J, Thorwesten L, Bork H, et al. Is prophylactic bracing of the ankle cost effective? Orthopedics 1996;19(5):405–14.

46. Tsikopoulos K, Sidiropoulos K, Kitridis D, et al. Do external supports improve dynamic balance in patients with chronic ankle instability? A network meta-analysis. Clin Orthop Relat Res 2020;478(2):359–77.

47. Hals TM, Sitler MR, Mattacola CG. Effect of a semi-rigid ankle stabilizer on performance in persons with functional ankle instability. J Orthop Sports Phys Ther 2000;30:552–6.

48. Jerosch J, Thorwesten L, Frebel T, et al. Influence of external stabilizing devices of the ankle on sport-specific capabilities. Knee Surg Sports Traumatol Arthrosc 1997;5(1):50–7.

49. Gross MT, Clemence LM, Cox BD, et al. Effect of ankle orthoses on functional performance for individuals with recurrent lateral ankle sprains. J Orthop Sports Phys Ther 1997;25:245–52.

50. Wiley JP, Nigg BM. The effect of an ankle orthosis on ankle range of motion and performance. J Orthop Sports Phys Ther 1996;23(6):362–9.

51. Jerosch J, Schoppe R. Midterm effects of ankle joint supports on sensomotor and sport-specific capabilities. Knee Surg Sports Traumatol Arthrosc 2000;8:252–9.

52. Rosenbaum D, Kamps N, Bosch K, et al. The influence of external ankle braces on subjective and objective parameters of performance in a sports-related agility course. Knee Surg Sports Traumatol Arthrosc 2005;13:419–25.

53. Mann B, Gruber AH, Murphy SP, et al. The influence of ankle braces on functional performance tests and ankle joint range of motion. J Sport Rehabil 2019;28(8): 817–23.

54. Gross MT, Everts JR, Roberson SE, et al. Effect of Donjoy Ankle Ligament Protector and Aircast Sport-Stirrup orthoses on functional performance. J Orthop Sports Phys Ther 1994;19(3):150–6.

55. Camacho LD, Roward ZT, Deng Y, et al. Surgical management of lateral ankle instability in athletes. J Athl Train 2019;54(6):639–49.

56. Hermanns C, Coda R, Cheema S, et al. Review of variability in rehabilitation protocols after lateral ankle ligament surgery. Kans J Med 2020;13:152–9.

57. Pearce CJ, Tourne Y, Zellers J, et al. Rehabilitation after anatomical ankle ligament repair or reconstruction. Knee Surg Sports Traumatol Arthrosc 2016;24(4): 1130–9.

58. Zhao Dubuc Y, Mazzone B, Yoder AJ, et al. Ankle sprain bracing solutions and future design consideration for civilian and military use. Expert Rev Med Devices 2022;19(2):113–22.

59. Cusimano MD, Faress A, Luong WP, et al. Factors affecting ankle support device usage in young basketball players. J Clin Med 2013;2(2):22–31.
60. Janssen K, Van Den Berg A, Van Mechelen W, et al. User survey of 3 ankle braces in soccer, volleyball, and running: which brace fits best? J Athl Train 2017;52(8):730–7.
61. Klem NR, Wild CY, Williams SA, et al. Effect of external ankle support on ankle and knee biomechanics during the cutting maneuver in basketball players. Am J Sports Med 2017;45(3):685–91.
62. McGuine TA, Brooks A, Hetzel S. The effect of lace-up ankle braces on injury rates in high school basketball players. Am J Sports Med 2011;39(9):1840–8.
63. Denton JM, Waldhelm A, Hacke JD, et al. Clinician recommendations and perceptions of factors associated with ankle brace use. Sports Health 2015;7(3):267–9.

Disease-Specific Finite element Analysis of the Foot and Ankle

Hamed Malakoutikhah, PhD[a],*, Leonard Daniel Latt, MD, PhD[b]

KEYWORDS

- Finite-element modeling • Computational studies • Clinical implications
- Foot and ankle disorders • Pathomechanics • Surgical procedures

KEY POINTS

- Finite element (FE) analysis has been used both to investigate the pathomechanics of foot and ankle disorders and to evaluate the effectiveness of various surgical procedures.
- In comparison to experimental methods, FE analysis has the advantages of consistency in results, the ability to parameterize different aspects of the model, and the capability to precisely measure variables that are difficult or impossible to measure experimentally.
- Parameters calculated from FE models have been widely used to make predictions about their biomechanical correlates, for example, joint contact pressures, bone stress, plantar pressures, and ligament stresses can be used to determine the risk of developing osteoarthritis, fractures, plantar ulceration, and ligament degeneration, respectively.

INTRODUCTION

Finite element (FE) analysis is a computational modeling technique in which a system of algebraic equations is used to calculate the displacements, strains, stresses, and forces in a geometrically complex model. The principal inputs to the model consist of the model geometry, material properties, loading, and boundary conditions (constraints). FE analysis has frequently been used in medicine to design medical devices and analyze the effectiveness of surgical procedures. It possesses several advantages in comparison to experimental methods such as consistency in results, the ability to parameterize different aspects of the model, and the capability to quantify kinetic and kinematic variables that cannot be measured externally. The main disadvantage of FE analysis is the substantial time that is required to develop each model. Accordingly, most foot and ankle FE studies rely on a model built from a single subject, which

[a] Department of Aerospace and Mechanical Engineering, University of Arizona, 1130 North Mountain Avenue, Tucson, AZ 85721, USA; [b] Department of Orthopaedic Surgery, University of Arizona, 1501 N. Campbell Ave, Suite 8401, Tucson, AZ, 85724 USA
* Corresponding author.
E-mail address: hamedmalak@arizona.edu

Foot Ankle Clin N Am 28 (2023) 155–172
https://doi.org/10.1016/j.fcl.2022.10.007
foot.theclinics.com

may limit the external validity of their findings. In contrast, a few foot and ankle FE studies have used multiple samples but to do so have had to limit the complexity of the model through simplifying assumptions or by scaling back to include only a limited number of anatomic structures.

An FE model consists of a mesh of FEs that are arranged in the three-dimensional geometry of the object of interest. The three-dimensional geometry of tissue and bone is usually reconstructed from MRI or computed tomography (CT) scan images, and each tissue is then modeled as a "mesh" of FEs in FE software (**Fig. 1**). Owing to the complexity of the foot and ankle, several simplifying assumptions are used in the assignment of material properties, loading, and boundary conditions. For example, ligaments that are capable of transferring tension but not compression are often simulated using tension-only truss or spring elements, and the pull of the muscle-tendon unit on the bone are often modeled simply as a force vector acting at the tendon insertion onto bone. The material properties of each of the tissues are usually chosen to follow the idealized behavior of a linear elastic, hyperelastic, or viscoelastic solid. Several review articles have focused on the technical details of developing FE models of the foot and ankle.[1,2]

In FE studies, the biomechanical impacts of foot disorders and surgical procedures are analyzed by monitoring changes in biomechanical parameters. The parameters chosen depend on the disease/disorder/deformity under study. Many of these biomechanical parameters have direct physiologic correlates. For example, plantar peak pressure is used to assess the risk of plantar ulceration, increases in joint contact pressure are correlated with the development of osteoarthritis, increased ligament tension is correlated with ligament degeneration, and increased bone stress is used as an index for the development of stress fractures.

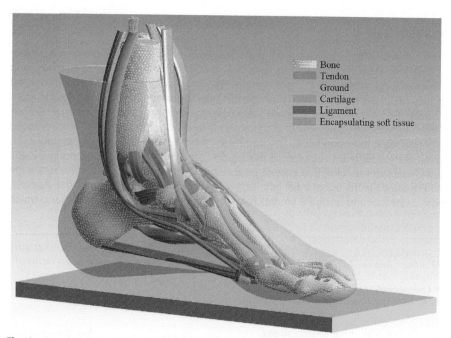

Bone
Tendon
Ground
Cartilage
Ligament
Encapsulating soft tissue

Fig. 1. A typical finite-element model of the foot and ankle.

The anatomic complexity of the foot and ankle precludes the use of a single comprehensive FE model for all analyses; instead, the features of the model are usually chosen to include only those needed to answer a specific question. Thus, one way to characterize the different FE models of the foot that have been developed is by the disorder or disease that is addressed. The models can then be further subdivided as to those that are addressing foot mechanics or pathomechanics or those that are evaluating a certain treatment. In this review, we focus on providing an overview of FE studies of foot and ankle disorders, including both those that are aimed at understanding the pathomechanics and those that seek to evaluate the effectiveness of various surgical procedures. Moreover, where possible, we describe the potential clinical implications of each of these studies.

PROGRESSIVE COLLAPSING FOOT DEFORMITY

Progressive collapsing foot deformity (PCFD), also known as adult-acquired flatfoot deformity (AAFD) or posterior tibial tendon dysfunction (PTTD), is a complex three-dimensional deformity characterized by hindfoot valgus, forefoot abduction, and arch collapse.[3] PCFD resulting from degeneration of the active and passive soft tissue stabilizers of the foot[3] has been the subject of several published FE models. The deformity has been simulated either by reducing the stiffness[4,5] or removing[6,7] the plantar fascia, long plantar, short plantar, deltoid, spring, and talocalcaneal interosseous ligaments which are the primary passive stabilizers of the arch, and unloading the posterior tibial tendon (PTT) which is the primary active stabilizer of the arch. Most of the FE studies have used a single model derived from a neutrally aligned foot; in contrast, two studies have used patient-specific models reconstructed using the bones of PCFD patients.[5,8]

Pathomechanics

The role of soft tissue stabilizers on the kinematic and kinetic aspects of the foot has been examined by removing them one at a time and comparing the results with those of the normal and collapsed foot.[4,6,7,9,10] It has been shown that isolated failure of the plantar fascia, long plantar, short plantar, or spring ligament increases the load on the remaining ones.[4,6,9–11] This is particularly true for the plantar fascia. The plantar fascia has been reported to be the most important contributor to arch stability,[4,7,9] whereas the deltoid ligament and the spring ligament have been identified as the primary contributors to the prevention of hindfoot valgus and forefoot abduction, respectively.[7] Isolated failure of PTT has been shown to have little effect on foot alignment,[10] but it alters load transfer of the medial column[12] and increases the force in the deltoid and spring ligaments.[10] The ability of the PTT to restore foot alignment has been investigated by gradually increasing the force within the PTT in a collapsed foot with attenuated ligaments and comparing foot alignment angles to the normal foot.[10] In this study, when simulating the collapsed foot, the tibia was unconstrained in all planes except axial translation which created the degrees of freedom needed to allow for relative internal rotation of the talus and valgus of the calcaneus resulting in greater deformity than other PCFD models. The results suggest that the PTT can restore alignment in a collapsed foot, primarily by reducing hindfoot valgus and forefoot abduction, but at a higher load, which could cause its injury over time.

The impact of ligament failure and subsequent flatfoot on joint contact mechanics has also been assessed using FE analysis. A recent study showed that collapsing the foot leads to an increase in contact pressure in the subtalar, calcaneocuboid, and tibiotalar joints but a decrease in contact pressure in the talonavicular joint.[13] Failure of the spring ligament has been found to be the primary cause of increased contact pressure in the subtalar and calcaneocuboid joints, whereas deltoid ligament failure is the main contributor to increased contact pressure in the medial naviculocuneiform, first tarsometatarsal, and tibiotalar joints.

Surgical Procedures

FE models of the foot have also been used to predict the biomechanical consequences of flatfoot surgical procedures including bony osteotomies, tendon transfers, and ligament reconstructions, and arthrodeses. Lateral column lengthening (opening wedge osteotomy of the body of the calcaneus) was shown to offload the medial forefoot while increasing calcaneocuboid joint contact force and unevenly straining plantar structures.[14] The shape of graft used in lateral column lengthening was also investigated using a patient-specific FE model. In comparison to triangular grafts, the rectangular graft was reported to provide a higher degree of correction but unevenly distributed pressure in the calcaneocuboid and talonavicular joints.[8] The medializing calcaneal osteotomy was simulated by translating the posterior tuberosity of the calcaneus medially by 5 to 10 mm.[5,14] This osteotomy was found to produce the most change in hindfoot alignment angle[14] and significantly improve the alignment of the medial column of the foot.[5]

The triple arthrodesis has been simulated by using bonded contacts at the talocalcaneal, talonavicular, and calcaneocuboid joints in a simplified foot model that included the tibia, talus, calcaneus, navicular, and cuboid.[15] The results showed that the triple arthrodesis reduces cortical bone surface strain and shifts stress distribution from the medial to the lateral side with a more even distribution than isolated subtalar arthrodesis. Double hindfoot arthrodesis (talonavicular and subtalar joints) was compared with isolated subtalar or talonavicular arthrodesis in a simplified model with four ligaments, no tibia, and no encapsulating soft tissue.[16] Isolated talonavicular arthrodesis was found to be superior to isolated subtalar and almost equivalent to triple arthrodesis due to its significant stress reduction on both the plantar fascia and the spring ligament.

Ligament reconstructions have been examined in two FE models. A recent study showed that nonanatomic reconstructions of the spring ligament provide more restoration of foot alignment than anatomic reconstructions, but neither can restore talonavicular and calcaneocuboid joint contact pressures.[17] Biomechanical analysis of several approaches to deltoid ligament reconstruction was performed using an FE model of the ankle including six bony structures and nine principal ligaments surrounding the ankle joint complex.[18] The results showed that no reconstruction could completely restore ankle alignment, but the reconstructions described by Kitaoka and Deland (tunneled allograft reconstruction from the medial malleolus to the medial cuneiform and from the medial malleolus to the talus, respectively) have advantages in terms of rotational stability and ligament stress when compared with the reconstructions describe by Wiltberger and Hintermann (tunneled allograft reconstruction from the medial malleolus to the navicular).

Subtalar arthroeresis, in which an implant is placed into the sinus tarsi to prevent physiologic eversion,[19] has also been evaluated in a recent FE study.[20] It was found that a customized sinus tarsi implant raises navicular height, relieves strain on the plantar navicular ligament, and lateralizes the rearfoot load transfer pathway. However, it causes stress concentration at the sinus tarsi.

HALLUX VALGUS

A few patient-specific models with first metatarsophalangeal joint valgus and first tarsometatarsal varus have been used to investigate the biomechanical effects of hallux valgus (HV) (bunion) on the foot.[21] However, most of the studies that have evaluated the consequences of HV correction have used normal foot models.[22–25]

Pathomechanics

Using a single-subject FE model that represented a severe HV foot with a hallux valgus angle of 23° and an intermetatarsal angle of 14° (**Fig. 2**A), it was found that increased metatarsal stress and decreased first ray load-carrying capacity are two biomechanical consequences of HV.[26] In addition, several potential causes of the deformity have been investigated in FE studies, including both acquired and hereditary causes. The effect of generalized ligament laxity on the development of HV was examined as the intrinsic cause of HV.[27] It was shown that generalized ligament laxity can cause HV by reducing metatarsophalangeal joint loading. The geometry and sexual dimorphism of the proximal phalanx of the hallux were also investigated as important factors in the formation of bunions. According to a study involving ten different FE models of the hallux in the

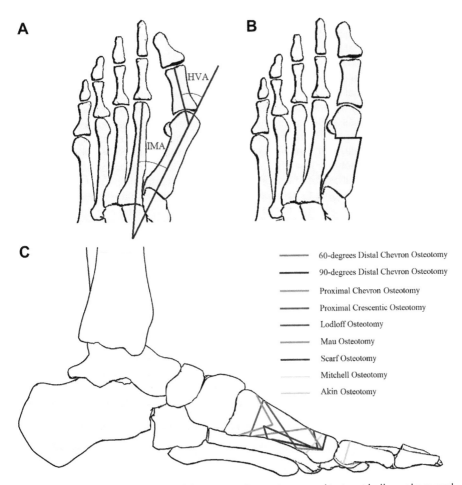

A

HVA

IMA

B

C

------- 60-degrees Distal Chevron Osteotomy
------- 90-degrees Distal Chevron Osteotomy
------- Proximal Chevron Osteotomy
------- Proximal Crescentic Osteotomy
------- Lodloff Osteotomy
------- Mau Osteotomy
------- Scarf Osteotomy
------- Mitchell Osteotomy
------- Akin Osteotomy

Fig. 2. (*A*) Hallux valgus deformity, (*B*) metatarsal osteotomy used to treat hallux valgus, and (*C*) different types of metatarsal osteotomy (HVA: Hallux valgus angle; IMA: intermetatarsal angle).

toe-off stage,[21] the difference in length between the medial and lateral sides of the hallux is greater in women, exposing it to more stresses that could cause the hallux to rotate toward a more relaxed position, making it more prone to develop HV.

On the other hand, numerous FE studies have assumed that HV is more commonly acquired than hereditary, and that footwear plays a significant role in the progression of HV. To verify this hypothesis, a recent study compared the stress concentration in FE models of the first metatarsophalangeal joint of fossil remains of bear-footed Homo naledi, which is an ideal model for non-shoe-wearing individuals, with that of contemporary shoe-wearing wrestlers.[28] Their findings showed that stress concentration is much higher in a simulated shoe-wearing condition than in a barefooted condition, which may contribute to the formation of bunions. The limitations of these models were that they included only the first ray and excluded ligaments and tendons, which could alter the stress distribution between joints and ligaments. The stress concentration in the first metatarsophalangeal joint is found to be even higher in the foot with a high-heeled support.[29]

Surgical Procedures

Of the many first tarsometatarsal osteotomies used in the treatment of HV (**Fig. 2**B, C), only the chevron osteotomy has been studied using FE analysis. Three studies have been conducted which seek to determine the optimal angle of the chevron and displacement of the osteotomy.[22–24] One study that used a two-dimensional FE model of the first metatarsal compared the traditional sixty-degree chevron to a ninety-degree chevron osteotomy and found improved mechanical bonding, owing to stronger compressive stresses at the osteotomy site and weaker shear stresses that tend to slide the two bone parts apart.[22] Stress in the metatarsals and stress concentration in the first metatarsophalangeal joint were also found to be minimized when the degree of displacement of ninety-degree chevron osteotomy is 4 mm.[24] Despite the numerous benefits of metatarsal osteotomies for treating HV, the shortening of the first metatarsal after the surgery is thought to cause postoperative transfer metatarsalgia. A maximum of 6-mm shortening length was found to be within a safe range for chevron osteotomy, with allowable changes in forefoot loading pattern during the push-off phase of gait.[23]

Arthrodesis of the first tarsometatarsal joint (Lapidus) which is used to treat severe HV or first tarsometatarsal arthritis has been examined in several studies. An FE study simulated tarsometatarsal arthrodesis by resecting parts of the first metatarsal and cuneiform and assigning a bone graft with the same stiffness as adjacent bones.[30] They found that Lapidus reduced the medial excursion of the first metatarsal head and restored the load-bearing function of the first ray. However, it was also found to cause increased plantar, navicocuneiform and fifth tarsometatarsal joint contact pressures, as well as increased metatarsal stresses which could increase the risk of developing stress fractures or osteoarthritis.[25] In tarsometatarsal arthrodesis, the relative motion of tarsometatarsal joints can be constrained using screws or fixation plates. In a three segment FE model consisting of the first tarsometatarsal and the cuneiform, Yu and colleagues simulated plate fixation of the first tarsometatarsal joint fracture-dislocation using two different implants, a locking plate and a five-hole 1/4 tubular plate.[31] They found that using the 1/4 tubular plate is preferable because it results in less displacement of the articular surface and less stress on the locking plate.

HALLUX RIGIDUS

Patients with hallux rigidus (HR), or osteoarthritis of the first metatarsophalangeal joint, are troubled by both the pain and the stiffness that occur at this joint. For this reason, it is crucial to consider both joint mobility and stress when modeling this disorder. Most studies of HR have relied on a simplified foot model that only includes the first ray.[32] HR has been simulated by simply restricting the degrees of freedom of the hallux. For example, Budhabhatti and colleagues increased the stiffness of the connectors placed at the metatarsophalangeal and interphalangeal joints to simulate joint immobility.[33]

Pathomechanics

An FE study has examined tightness of the plantar fascia, contracture of the flexor hallucis brevis muscle, and mismatch of the articular surfaces as potential causes of abnormal stress on the first metatarsophalangeal joint using an FE model of the first ray.[32] Their findings showed that an increase in plantar fascia tension is the primary contributor to the abnormal joint stress and the progression of HR. Using another FE model of the first ray, it was also shown that simulated HR leads to high plantar pressures beneath the first ray.[33] The limitations of these models, including the use of a healthy foot model, the modeling of only the first ray, and the lack of the sesamoids, may have had an impact on the magnitude of predicted values.

Surgical Procedures

The same model[33] was used to investigate the biomechanical consequences of first metatarsophalangeal arthrodesis, which is a classic pain-relieving surgery used to treat HR and severe HV. To simulate this procedure, the joint was fixed in the conventional dorsiflexion angle of 36°, whereas the valgus angle was kept at 15°. The results showed a significant increase in hallux stress, but a decrease in plantar pressure beneath the first ray.

Metatarsophalangeal joint replacement (arthroplasty) is another surgical option for the treatment of severe HR. Joint arthroplasty has been shown to significantly increase strain and stress in the first metatarsal and proximal phalange at the toe-off stage, which may be the cause of postoperative complications.[34] This is especially true when arthroplasty has been performed with the Swanson implant rather than the Tornier implant. Although a complete anatomic model of the foot was used for this study, the accuracy of the findings could be affected by the use of a coarse mesh with some skew elements and by the neglect of the pre-stress in the implants as a result of the deformation the foot model experienced during the analysis stage.

LESSER TOE DEFORMITIES

As lesser toe deformities (hammer toe, mallet toe, and claw toe deformities; **Fig. 3**) cause hyperextension and hyperflexion of the metatarsophalangeal, proximal, and/ or distal interphalangeal joints of the second to fifth toes, FE studies have focused on biomechanical changes in these joints before[35] and after[36,37] surgical corrections.

Pathomechanics

To investigate the impact of hammer toe deformity on internal stresses during gait, a patient-specific foot model was created from a diabetic neuropathic volunteer with a hammer toe in the left foot and no deformity in the right foot.[35] The results revealed that the hammer toe increases stress in the metatarsals and proximal phalanges as well as plantar pressure beneath the forefoot, potentially leading to forefoot ulcers.

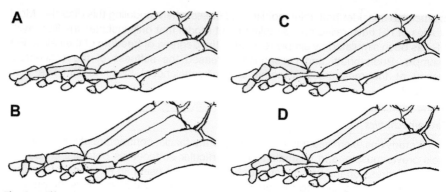

Fig. 3. Different types of lesser toe deformities: (*A*) normal, (*B*) mallet toe, (*C*) hammer toe, and (*D*) claw toe.

Surgical Procedures

Lesser toe deformities can be treated with a variety of techniques, including flexor digitorum longus (FDL) and flexor digitorum brevis (FDB) tendon transfers and proximal interphalangeal joint arthrodesis. FDL and FDB tendon transfers, simulated by transferring tendon forces to the dorsal aspect of proximal phalanges, have been shown to reduce stress and dorsal displacement of the proximal phalanx, as well as dorsiflexion of the metatarsophalangeal joint, primarily in the second and third toes.[36] It was also shown that there is a biomechanical advantage to performing FDL or FDB tendon transfer rather than proximal interphalangeal joint arthrodesis in terms of stress and strain in the second metatarsal, which reduces the risk of metatarsalgia or stress fracture.[37] The same model, constructed from a healthy foot with no deformities, was used in both of these studies. Both were also analyzed in the toe-off phase of the gait cycle when all stresses and displacements in the first ray are at their maximum.

ANKLE ARTHRITIS

Most of the FE models used to study ankle arthritis have included only the bones adjacent to the ankle joint.[38–41] In contrast, a few models have attempted to model the whole foot and ankle complex.[42]

Pathomechanics

Variation in joint contact stresses has been proposed as a metric of mechano-stimulus abnormality, plausibly correlating with degeneration propensity.[42] Osteoarthritis secondary to altered joint contact stresses is particularly true for the ankle joint as it is rarely a site of idiopathic primary osteoarthritis. According to a recent FE study, failure of the deltoid ligament combined with attenuation of the plantar ligaments is the primary cause of valgus malalignment of the ankle and subsequent increased contact pressure in the joint.[13]

Surgical Procedures

Several FE models have studied ankle arthrodesis (AA) and total ankle arthroplasty (TAA) in the treatment of tibiotalar osteoarthritis. AA has been simulated either by bonding the talus and tibia together[43] or by constraining joint motion with screws, plates, or pins.[38–40] The FE models have been used to evaluate the biomechanical effects of AA on the whole foot and ankle,[43] as well as the type, material, number, and configuration of screws used in this procedure.[38,40,41,44] It was shown that AA results in an increase in peak plantar pressure, contact forces in the naviculocuneiform, tarsometatarsal, and talonavicular joints, and stress in the second and third metatarsals.[43] By simulating the tibiotalar interface with Coulomb frictional and frictionless contacts one at a time, an FE study predicted better initial stability for AA when the joint contours are preserved rather than resected to produce flat surfaces.[44] The three-screw construct with fully threaded screws has been shown to provide increased mechanical stability and lower micromotion at the tibiotalar interface, compared with the two-screw construct with partially threaded (lag) screws.[38–40] It was also found that screw configurations with the posteromedial home-run screw avoid collision and have lower micromotion on the articular surface than those with the posterolateral home-run screw.[41]

TAA has been modeled in four FEA studies.[45] The questions posed in these studies have varied from forces and stresses in foot tissues to the initial micromotion of prosthesis components. TAA has been simulated using bonded contacts between the tibial and talar components and the cut surfaces of the tibia and talus in two-component prostheses,[46] and inserting the mobile bearing to slide between the tibial and talar components in three-component prostheses.[45] The results of an FE analysis of three-component TAA demonstrated that forces in the surrounding ligaments and contact pressures on both the talar and the tibial surfaces that articulate with the mobile bearing are within corresponding physiologic ranges during the stance phase of gait.[47] Another study found an increase in talus, first, and fourth metatarsal peak stress, as well as a decrease in intermediate cuneiform and calcaneus peak stress as a result of TAA.[46] In addition, an FE analysis revealed that the stress in the medial cuneonavicular joint, the second, and third metatarsals, and forces transmitted from the first ray are all affected by TAA.[45] One of the most serious complications after TAA is implant loosening, which is commonly associated with increased initial micromotion.[48] Among most commonly used TAA devices, Mobility and Salto were found to have the largest micromotion of tibial and talar components, respectively. It was also shown that any initial implant misalignment increases the risk of TAA failure by causing more implant-bone micromotion and bone strains.

The biomechanical impacts of TAA and AA were also compared using FE analysis.[49] In this study, the relative motion between the tibia and talus was constrained using a tie connection to simulate the AA, but the bones were free to move relatively in the implanted ankle prosthesis (STAR) used to simulate the TAA. The results showed that TAA provides a more acceptable plantar pressure distribution, but it also causes higher contact pressure, occurring in the medial cuneonavicular joint. However, neither surgery was able to restore normal force transmission through the foot.

ANKLE FRACTURE

FE analysis has been used to investigate both ankle fractures (medial,[50] lateral, and posterior malleolar fractures[51] and plafond (pilon) fractures[52] (fractures of the tibiotalar articular surface)) (**Fig. 4**). Most of the FE models used to study ankle fractures have only included the bones around the ankle joint.

Pathomechanics

Most of the FE ankle fracture pathomechanical studies have focused on posterior malleolar fractures.[51,53,54] In these studies, variations in ankle joint contact pressure have been used to assess the risk of osteoarthritis. The angle between the fracture line and the vertical axis on sagittal reconstruction images, known as the sagittal angle (see

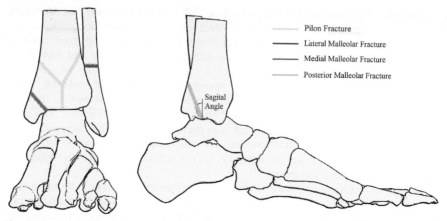

Pilon Fracture
Lateral Malleolar Fracture
Medial Malleolar Fracture
Posterior Malleolar Fracture

Sagital
Angle

Fig. 4. The most common ankle fractures.

Fig. 4), has been used as a measure of the relative height of fracture fragments. It was shown that the contact pressure is higher in the smaller sagittal angles.[53] In addition, the ankle joint contact pressure was found to be significantly increased by the intra-articular impacted fragment in the cartilage and subchondral bone in the region of posterior malleolus, potentially leading to posttraumatic osteoarthritis in the ankle joint.[54]

The effects of plafond fracture on ankle joint contact mechanics have been investigated by comparing the contact stress in the fractured ankles and the intact contralateral ankles using patient-specific FE models of 11 ankle pairs from tibial plafond fracture patients. It was shown that due to the presence of residual incongruities, fractured ankles have higher peak contact stresses that are less uniform and eccentrically located, predisposing the joint to posttraumatic osteoarthritis.[52] Additionally, fractured ankles had more area with high contact stress exposure and less area with low exposure compared with intact ankles.

Surgical Procedures

The effectiveness of two common fixation techniques for the treatment of transverse, oblique, and vertical medial malleolar fractures, the screw fixation and the plate fixation, was compared using FE analysis.[50] The FE model only included the distal tibia, which was fixed in all degrees of freedom on the proximal part and loaded with 700 N on the medial malleolar joint surface. The results showed that for oblique and vertical medial malleolar fractures, the stress in the tibia surrounding the screw in the 4.0-mm cancellous screw fixation is higher than the stress in the tibia surrounding the plate in the locking compression plate fixation, but there is no difference for transverse fractures. This suggests that, in transverse fractures, the traditional cancellous screw fixation is sufficient to prevent bone destruction and provide stable fixation without the need for the locking compression plate fixation.

Approaches to reduction and fixation of posterior malleolar fractures were evaluated using two FE models of the tibia. Half of the body weight was placed on the fracture fragment, whereas the proximal end of the tibia was fixed in all directions. The stress in the tibia surrounding the screws and relative fracture displacement in the posterior-anterior and anterior-posterior screw fixation techniques were reported to be higher than those surrounding the plate in the posterior buttress plate fixation technique.[55] Owing to higher fracture step-off and bone stress values, the reduction maintained by the posterior-anterior and anterior-posterior screws had a high tendency of fixation loss and bone cut-through, respectively. Furthermore, it has been reported that a larger posterior malleolar fracture causes more relative fracture displacement, necessitating a more stable fixation construct.[56]

SYNDESMOTIC ANKLE INJURY

Syndesmotic ankle injury (SAI), or high ankle sprain, is a common disorder involving the ligaments that connect the fibula to the tibia distally and thus function to maintain the ankle mortice. Syndesmotic injuries have been modeled in four FE studies.[57–60] Most of these have simulated SAI by simply removing the anterior and posterior inferior tibiofibular ligaments, the interosseous tibiofibular ligament, and a portion of the distal interosseous membrane closest to the tibiotalar joint.

Pathomechanics

The biomechanical effects of SAI have been investigated using one FE model of the foot and ankle.[57] It was found that SAI reduces contact forces between the talus and fibula, increases the displacement at the lower extremity of the tibia and fibula, and increases tibiotalar joint contact force. The absence of cartilage, the representation of bones as rigid objects, the exclusion of the midfoot and forefoot, and the use of simplified screw geometry were all limitations of this model.

Surgical Procedures

The gold standard for the treatment of SAI is a rigid fixation with screws or dynamic fixation with suture-button devices, which function to secure the syndesmotic relationship while the ligaments heal. Screw fixation of SAI was found to effectively stabilize syndesmotic diastasis by increasing the crural interosseous membrane stress and reducing the tibia and fibula displacement at the lower extremity.[57–60] However, because of the variations in stress distribution around the ankle and the reduction in joint range of motion caused by this procedure, the screws should be removed as soon as the injury heals. There is no FE study that has compared rigid to dynamic fixation techniques.

Several FE studies have been conducted on the biomechanical impact of number, diameter, position, material, and diameter of the syndesmotic screw, as well as the number of penetrated cortical bones.[58–60] Although there is no consensus on whether to use tricortical or quadricortical fixation, most studies have found that the use of 4.5 mm screws at a level of 20 to 25 mm above the ankle results in less syndesmosis widening and stress in the screws and adjacent bones, stabilizing the syndesmosis more effectively.

PLANTAR FASCIITIS

Plantar fasciitis (PF), a degenerative disorder of the insertion of the plantar fascia onto the calcaneus, has been examined in several FEA studies from 2006 to 2022. Four of these studies focused on pathomechanics[29,61–63] and five on the treatment of PF.[6,7,10,64,65] Most of the studies have modeled the plantar fascia using tension-only elements such as spring[10] or truss elements.[29,61–63] However, a few studies used linear elastic[29,61–63] or hyperelastic[65] isotropic solid elements which have the advantage of maintaining the anatomic geometry in the model, but has the disadvantage of potentially allowing the transmission of bending moments and compressive forces within the ligaments.

Pathomechanics

The biomechanical causes and effects of PF and the role of the heel spur have been examined in several FE studies.[29,61–63] An FE analysis of the female foot while wearing high heels revealed that elevation of the hindfoot with an arch-supporting insole results in a decrease in strain on the plantar fascia, which could be used as a treatment strategy for PF.[29] The optimal insole, in which the thickness of the insole toward the heel was varied between 1 and 3 cm in different positions, was found to reduce plantar fascia strain and stress by approximately 32% and 14%, respectively.[61] However, a recent FE study questioned the therapeutic benefit of high heels in the treatment of PF by demonstrating that the strain on the plantar fascia increases as the heel is raised from 3 to 7 cm.[62] The Achilles tendon can also be lengthened or tension relieved as a treatment option for PF. Additionally, a decrease in Achilles tendon force was found to reduce tension in the plantar fascia.[63] It also points to Achilles tendon tightness as a risk factor for PF.

Surgical Procedures

Partial plantar fasciotomy (cutting partway across the plantar fascia) is commonly used to treat PF refractory to conservative treatment. It is thought to stimulate healing of the plantar fascia. Where complete fascial release is simulated by removing the whole plantar fascia,[6,10] partial fascia release is simulated by removing only the medial band of the plantar fascia.[64] Several FE studies investigated the effect of individual release of the plantar fascia on arch integrity. They found that partial and total plantar fascia releases have very little impact on arch height,[7,64] but do increase the strain and stress in the plantar ligaments,[6,10,64] spring ligament, and superficial deltoid ligament[10] as well as stress in the metatarsals,[64] potentially putting the foot at risk of arch instability over time.[6,7,10,64]

Taping is a noninvasive treatment of PF in runners. The biomechanical impact of two different taping methods, low-dye taping and fascia taping, on plantar fascia tension during running was compared using FE analysis.[65] Fascia taping, as opposed to low-dye taping, was found to be very effective in reducing plantar fascia strain and increasing navicular height.

DIABETIC FOOT ULCERATION

Diabetic foot ulceration (DFU) occurs commonly in individuals with longstanding diabetes mellitus complicated by peripheral neuropathy. The development of plantar ulceration is multifactorial and likely related to the loss of protective sensation combined with the altered mechanical environment of the foot secondary to decreased lower-limb muscle strength,[66] increased plantar soft tissue stiffness,[67] foot deformity, and vascular dysregulation. FE analysis has been used to assess the biomechanical causes of DFU, as well as the effectiveness of various treatments.

Pathomechanics

The pathomechanics of DFU have been evaluated in FE models that simulate the mechanical properties of the diabetic foot by increasing the stiffness of the plantar soft tissues.[68,69] It was shown that DFU may be initiated internally from the lateral sesamoid associated with the first metatarsal head, where von Mises stress is maximum, and progress upwards to the outermost skin level.[70] Sensitivity analysis of soft tissue properties found that a fivefold increase in soft tissue stiffness causes a 7% increase in metatarsal stresses and a 35% increase in peak plantar pressure, potentially increasing the risk of plantar ulceration.[68] Reduced intrinsic and extrinsic muscle forces were also found to increase tissue and bone internal stresses, and negatively affect plantar pressure distribution.[71] This suggests a potential for therapeutic exercise in helping to prevent the formation of DFU.

Treatment

Accommodative insoles (those that are designed to evenly distribute and attenuate pressure across the foot) made from multiple layers of different foam of varying density have been used to reduce the risk of plantar ulceration. The efficiency of total contact insoles with three layers (PPT, Microcel Puff, and Thermocork) in stress reduction and redistribution was confirmed using FE analysis, where the foot with a total contact insole has lower plantar peak stresses than a regular flat insole.[72] Using a combined FE and Taguchi method (a product optimization method used to improve the quality of manufactured goods), the most important design factors in the design of arch-conforming insoles for peak pressure reduction were found to be the custom-molded shape and insole stiffness, rather than the thickness of the midsole and insole.[73] FE analysis was also used to optimize custom-made insoles with a cutout under the ulcer site in terms of three hole-geometry offloading parameters.[74] Holes with a large offloading depth and radius, as well as a relatively small radius of curvature, were found to optimally reduce heel loads in the soft tissues surrounding high-risk areas without causing edge effects.

FEA has also been used to confirm the effectiveness of using complaint midsole materials to offload specific regions of the foot. Two FE studies used softer plugs inserted into a monolithic total contact insole under the metatarsal heads and found lower peak plantar pressure than with the insole alone.[75] Pressure-relieving insoles with layered modular insoles that include eight layers of small cushions have also been evaluated and were shown to redistribute plantar pressure and lower peak pressures more effectively than traditional arch-conforming insoles.[69]

SUMMARY

FEA is a computational modeling technique that can be used to quantify parameters that are difficult or impossible to measure externally in a geometrically complex structure such as the foot and ankle. It has been used to improve our understanding of the pathomechanics and to evaluate proposed treatments for several disorders, including PCFD, HV, HR, PF, SAI, DFU, ankle arthritis, ankle fracture, and lesser toe deformities. The assumptions made for each model depend on the question it is intended to answer and must be taken into account in evaluating the results of the modeling effort.[76] Improvements in computing power will allow for the creation of increasingly sophisticated models that will better simulate actual biomechanics and pathomechanics and will thus play an increasingly important role in aiding treatment decision making.

CLINICS CARE POINTS

- The plantar fascia is the most important contributor to arch stability,[4,7,9] whereas the deltoid ligament and the spring ligament are the primary contributors to the prevention of hindfoot valgus and forefoot abduction, respectively.[7]
- Generalized ligament laxity can cause hallux valgus by reducing metatarsophalangeal joint loading.[27]

- An increase in plantar fascia tension is the primary contributor to the abnormal joint stress and the progression of hallux rigidus.[32]
- The hammer toe increases stress in the metatarsals and proximal phalanges as well as plantar pressure beneath the forefoot, potentially leading to forefoot ulcers.[35]
- Total ankle arthroplasty provides a more normal plantar pressure distribution compared with ankle arthrodesis.[49]
- Fractured ankles have higher peak contact stresses that are less uniform and eccentrically located, predisposing the joint to posttraumatic osteoarthritis.[52]
- Plantar fascia releases have very little impact on arch height,[7,64] but do increase the stress in the plantar ligaments,[6,10,64] spring ligament, and superficial deltoid ligament[10] as well as stress in the metatarsals,[64] potentially putting the foot at risk of arch instability over time.[6,7,10,64]

CONFLICT OF INTEREST STATEMENT

The authors have nothing to disclose.

REFERENCES

1. Morales-orcajo E, Bayod J, Estevam, et al. Computational Foot Modeling: Scope and Applications. Arch Comput Methods Eng 2016;23(3):389–416.
2. Behforootan S, Chatzistergos P, Naemi R, et al. Finite-element modelling of the foot for clinical application: A systematic review. Med Eng Phys 2017;39:1–11.
3. Myerson MS, Thordarson DB, Johnson JE, et al. Classification and Nomenclature: Progressive Collapsing Foot Deformity. Foot Ankle Int 2020;41(10):1271–6.
4. Iaquinto JM, Wayne JS. Computational model of the lower leg and foot/ankle complex: application to arch stability. J Biomech Eng 2010;132(2):021009.
5. Spratley EM, Matheis EA, Hayes CW, et al. Effects of Degree of Surgical Correction for Flatfoot Deformity in Patient-Specific Computational Models. Ann Biomed Eng 2015;43(8):1947–56.
6. Tao K, Ji WT, Wang DM, et al. Relative contributions of plantar fascia and ligaments on the arch static stability: a finite-element study. Biomed Tech (Berl) 2010;55(5):265–71.
7. Malakoutikhah H, Madenci E, Latt LD. The contribution of the ligaments in progressive collapsing foot deformity: A comprehensive computational study. J Orthop Res 2022;40(9):2209–21.
8. Wu J, Liu H, Xu C. Biomechanical Effects of Graft Shape for the Evans Lateral Column Lengthening Procedure: A Patient-Specific Finite-element Investigation. Foot Ankle Int 2022;43(3):404–13.
9. Cifuentes-De la Portilla C, Larrainzar-Garijo R, Bayod J. Analysis of the main passive soft tissues associated with adult acquired flatfoot deformity development: A computational modeling approach. J Biomech 2019;84:183–90.
10. Malakoutikhah H, Madenci E, Latt LD. A computational model of force within the ligaments and tendons in progressive collapsing foot deformity. J Orthop Res 2022;1–11.
11. Cheung JT, Nigg BM. Clinical Applications of Computational Simulation of Foot and Ankle. Sports Orthopaedics Traumatol 2008;23(4):264–71.
12. Wong DW, Wang Y, Leung AK, et al. Finite-element simulation on posterior tibial tendinopathy: Load transfer alteration and implications to the onset of pes planus. Clin Biomech 2018;51:10–6.

13. Malakoutikhah H, Madenci E, Latt LD. The impact of ligament tears on joint contact mechanics in progressive collapsing foot deformity: A finite-element study. Clin Biomech 2022;94:105630.

14. Iaquinto JM, Wayne JS. Effects of surgical correction for the treatment of adult acquired flatfoot deformity: a computational investigation. J Orthop Res 2011;29(7): 1047–54.

15. Chitsazan A, Herzog W, Rouhi G, et al. Alteration of Strain Distribution in Distal Tibia After Triple Arthrodesis: Experimental and Finite-element Investigations. J Med Biol Eng 2018;38:469–81.

16. Cifuentes-De la Portilla C, Larrainzar-Garijo R, Bayod J. Analysis of biomechanical stresses caused by hindfoot joint arthrodesis in the treatment of adult acquired flatfoot deformity: A finite-element study. Foot Ankle Surg 2020;26(4): 412–20.

17. Xu C, Li MQ, Wang C, et al. Nonanatomic versus anatomic techniques in spring ligament reconstruction: biomechanical assessment via a finite-element model. J Orthop Surg Res 2019;14(1):114.

18. Xu C, Zhang MY, Lei GH, et al. Biomechanical evaluation of tenodesis reconstruction in ankle with deltoid ligament deficiency: a finite-element analysis. Knee Surg Sports Traumatol Arthrosc 2012;20(9):1854–62.

19. Henry JK, Shakked R, Ellis SJ. Adult-Acquired Flatfoot Deformity. Foot Ankle Orthop 2019;4(1). 2473011418820847.

20. Wong DW, Wang Y, Niu W, et al. Finite-element analysis of subtalar joint arthroereisis on adult-acquired flexible flatfoot deformity using customised sinus tarsi implant. J Orthop Translat 2021;27:139–45.

21. Morales-Orcajo E, Bayod J, Becerro-de-Bengoa-Vallejo R, et al. Influence of first proximal phalanx geometry on hallux valgus deformity: a finite-element analysis. Med Biol Eng Comput 2015;53(7):645–53.

22. Matzaroglou C, Bougas P, Panagiotopoulos E, et al. Ninety-degree chevron osteotomy for correction of hallux valgus deformity: clinical data and finite-element analysis. Open Orthop J 2010;4:152–6.

23. Geng X, Shi J, Chen W, et al. Impact of first metatarsal shortening on forefoot loading pattern: a finite-element model study. BMC Musculoskelet Disord 2019; 20(1):625.

24. Zhang Q, Zhang Y, Huang J, et al. Effect of Displacement Degree of Distal Chevron Osteotomy on Metatarsal Stress: A Finite-element Method. Biology (Basel) 2022;11(1).

25. Wang Y, Li Z, Zhang M. Biomechanical study of tarsometatarsal joint fusion using finite-element analysis. Med Eng Phys 2014;36(11):1394–400.

26. Zhang Y, Awrejcewicz J, Szymanowska O, et al. Effects of severe hallux valgus on metatarsal stress and the metatarsophalangeal loading during balanced standing: A finite-element analysis. Comput Biol Med 2018;97:1–7.

27. Wong DW, Wang Y, Chen TL, et al. Finite-element Analysis of Generalized Ligament Laxity on the Deterioration of Hallux Valgus Deformity (Bunion). Front Bioeng Biotechnol 2020;8:571192.

28. Yu G, Fan Y, Fan Y, et al. The Role of Footwear in the Pathogenesis of Hallux Valgus: A Proof-of-Concept Finite-element Analysis in Recent Humans and Homo naledi. Front Bioeng Biotechnol 2020;8:648.

29. Yu J, Cheung JT, Fan Y, et al. Development of a finite-element model of female foot for high-heeled shoe design. Clin Biomech 2008;23(Suppl 1):S31–8.

30. Wai-Chi Wong D, Wang Y, Zhang M, et al. Functional restoration and risk of non-union of the first metatarsocuneiform arthrodesis for hallux valgus: A finite-element approach. J Biomech 2015;48(12):3142–8.

31. Yu X, Li WL, Pang QJ, et al. Finite-element analysis of locking plate and 1/4 tubular plate for first tarsometatarsal joint fracture-dislocation. J Int Med Res 2017;45(5):1528–34.

32. Flavin R, Halpin T, O'Sullivan R, et al. A finite-element analysis study of the metatarsophalangeal joint of the hallux rigidus. J Bone Joint Surg Br 2008;90(10): 1334–40.

33. Budhabhatti SP, Erdemir A, Petre M, et al. Finite-element modeling of the first ray of the foot: a tool for the design of interventions. J Biomech Eng 2007;129(5): 750–6.

34. Martinez Bocanegra MA, Bayod Lopez J, Vidal-Lesso A, et al. Structural interaction between bone and implants due to arthroplasty of the first metatarsophalangeal joint. Foot Ankle Surg 2019;25(2):150–7.

35. Moayedi M, Arshi AR, Salehi M, et al. Associations between changes in loading pattern, deformity, and internal stresses at the foot with hammer toe during walking; a finite-element approach. Comput Biol Med 2021;135:104598.

36. Garcia-Gonzalez A, Bayod J, Prados-Frutos JC, et al. Finite-element simulation of flexor digitorum longus or flexor digitorum brevis tendon transfer for the treatment of claw toe deformity. J Biomech 2009;42(11):1697–704.

37. Bayod J, Becerro de Bengoa Vallejo R, Losa Iglesias ME, et al. Stress at the second metatarsal bone after correction of hammertoe and claw toe deformity: a finite-element analysis using an anatomical model. J Am Podiatr Med Assoc 2013;103(4):260–73.

38. Bing F, Wei C, Liu P, et al. Biomechanical finite-element analysis of typical tibiotalar arthrodesis. Med Novel Technology Devices 2021;11:100087.

39. Anderson RT, Pacaccio DJ, Yakacki CM, et al. Finite-element analysis of a pseudoelastic compression-generating intramedullary ankle arthrodesis nail. J Mech Behav Biomed Mater 2016;62:83–92.

40. Alonso-Vazquez A, Lauge-Pedersen H, Lidgren L, et al. Initial stability of ankle arthrodesis with three-screw fixation. A finite-element analysis. Clin Biomech 2004;19(7):751–9.

41. Wang S, Yu J, Ma X, et al. Finite-element analysis of the initial stability of arthroscopic ankle arthrodesis with three-screw fixation: posteromedial versus posterolateral home-run screw. J Orthop Surg Res 2020;15(1):252.

42. Anderson DD, Goldsworthy JK, Shivanna K, et al. Intra-articular contact stress distributions at the ankle throughout stance phase-patient-specific finite-element analysis as a metric of degeneration propensity. Biomech Model Mechanobiol 2006;5(2–3):82–9.

43. Wang Y, Li Z, Wong DW, et al. Effects of Ankle Arthrodesis on Biomechanical Performance of the Entire Foot. PLoS One 2015;10(7):e0134340.

44. Vazquez AA, Lauge-Pedersen H, Lidgren L, et al. Finite-element analysis of the initial stability of ankle arthrodesis with internal fixation: flat cut versus intact joint contours. Clin Biomech 2003;18(3):244–53.

45. Wang Y, Li Z, Wong DW, et al. Finite-element analysis of biomechanical effects of total ankle arthroplasty on the foot. J Orthop Translat 2018;12:55–65.

46. Ozen M, Sayman O, Havitcioglu H. Modeling and stress analyses of a normal foot-ankle and a prosthetic foot-ankle complex. Acta Bioeng Biomech 2013; 15(3):19–27.

47. Reggiani B, Leardini A, Corazza F, et al. Finite-element analysis of a total ankle replacement during the stance phase of gait. J Biomech 2006;39(8):1435–43.

48. Sopher RS, Amis AA, Calder JD, et al. Total ankle replacement design and positioning affect implant-bone micromotion and bone strains. Med Eng Phys 2017; 42:80–90.

49. Wang Y, Wong DW, Tan Q, et al. Total ankle arthroplasty and ankle arthrodesis affect the biomechanics of the inner foot differently. Sci Rep 2019;9(1):13334.

50. Jiang D, Zhan S, Wang Q, et al. Biomechanical Comparison of Locking Plate and Cancellous Screw Techniques in Medial Malleolar Fractures: A Finite-element Analysis. J Foot Ankle Surg 2019;58(6):1138–44.

51. Alonso-Rasgado T, Jimenez-Cruz D, Karski M. 3-D computer modelling of malunited posterior malleolar fractures: effect of fragment size and offset on ankle stability, contact pressure and pattern. J Foot Ankle Res 2017;10:13.

52. Li W, Anderson DD, Goldsworthy JK, et al. Patient-specific finite-element analysis of chronic contact stress exposure after intraarticular fracture of the tibial plafond. J Orthop Res 2008;26(8):1039–45.

53. Guan M, Zhao J, Kuang Y, et al. Finite-element analysis of the effect of sagittal angle on ankle joint stability in posterior malleolus fracture: A cohort study. Int J Surg 2019;70:53–9.

54. Xie W, Lu H, Yuan Y, et al. A new finite-element model of intra-articular impacted fragment in posterior malleolar fractures: A technical note. Injury 2022;53(2): 784–8.

55. Anwar A, Hu Z, Adnan A, et al. Comprehensive biomechanical analysis of three clinically used fixation constructs for posterior malleolar fractures using cadaveric and finite-element analysis. Sci Rep 2020;10(1):18639.

56. Anwar A, Lv D, Zhao Z, et al. Finite-element analysis of the three different posterior malleolus fixation strategies in relation to different fracture sizes. Injury 2017; 48(4):825–32.

57. Liu Q, Zhang K, Zhuang Y, et al. Analysis of the stress and displacement distribution of inferior tibiofibular syndesmosis injuries repaired with screw fixation: a finite-element study. PLoS One 2013;8(12):e80236.

58. Goh TS, Lim BY, Lee JS, et al. Identification of Surgical Plan for Syndesmotic Fixation Procedure Based on Finite-element Method. Appl Sci 2020;10(12):4349.

59. Li H, Chen Y, Qiang M, et al. Computational biomechanical analysis of postoperative inferior tibiofibular syndesmosis: a modified modeling method. Comput Methods Biomech Biomed Engin 2018;21(5):427–35.

60. Er MS, Verim O, Altinel L, et al. Three-dimensional finite-element analysis used to compare six different methods of syndesmosis fixation with 3.5- or 4.5-mm titanium screws: a biomechanical study. J Am Podiatr Med Assoc 2013;103(3): 174–80.

61. Hsu YC, Gung YW, Shih SL, et al. Using an optimization approach to design an insole for lowering plantar fascia stress–a finite-element study. Ann Biomed Eng 2008;36(8):1345–52.

62. Wang M, Li S, Teo EC, et al. The Influence of Heel Height on Strain Variation of Plantar Fascia During High Heel Shoes Walking-Combined Musculoskeletal Modeling and Finite-element Analysis. Front Bioeng Biotechnol 2021;9:791238.

63. Cheung JT, Zhang M, An KN. Effect of Achilles tendon loading on plantar fascia tension in the standing foot. Clin Biomech 2006;21(2):194–203.

64. Cheung JT, An KN, Zhang M. Consequences of partial and total plantar fascia release: a finite-element study. Foot Ankle Int 2006;27(2):125–32.

65. Chen TL, Wong DW, Peng Y, et al. Prediction on the plantar fascia strain offload upon Fascia taping and Low-Dye taping during running. J Orthop Translat 2020; 20:113–21.
66. Andersen H, Poulsen PL, Mogensen CE, et al. Isokinetic muscle strength in long-term IDDM patients in relation to diabetic complications. Diabetes 1996;45(4): 440–5.
67. Gefen A, Megido-Ravid M, Azariah M, et al. Integration of plantar soft tissue stiffness measurements in routine MRI of the diabetic foot. Clin Biomech 2001;16(10): 921–5.
68. Cheung JT, Zhang M, Leung AK, et al. Three-dimensional finite-element analysis of the foot during standing–a material sensitivity study. J Biomech 2005;38(5): 1045–54.
69. Niu J. Arearch-conforming insoles agoodfit for diabetic foot? Insole customized design by using finite-element analysis. Hum Factors Man 2020;30(4):3030–310.
70. Chen WM, Lee T, Lee PV, et al. Effects of internal stress concentrations in plantar soft-tissue–A preliminary three-dimensional finite-element analysis. Med Eng Phys 2010;32(4):324–31.
71. Scarton A, Guiotto A, Malaquias T, et al. A methodological framework for detecting ulcers' risk in diabetic foot subjects by combining gait analysis, a new musculoskeletal foot model and a foot finite-element model. Gait Posture 2018;60: 279–85.
72. Chen WP, Ju CW, Tang FT. Effects of total contact insoles on the plantar stress redistribution: a finite-element analysis. Clin Biomech 2003;18(6):S17–24.
73. Cheung JT, Zhang M. Parametric design of pressure-relieving foot orthosis using statistics-based finite-element method. Med Eng Phys 2008;30(3):269–77.
74. Shaulian H, Gefen A, Solomonow-Avnon D, et al. Finite-element-based method for determining an optimal offloading design for treating and preventing heel ulcers. Comput Biol Med 2021;131:104261.
75. Actis RL, Ventura LB, Lott DJ, et al. Multi-plug insole design to reduce peak plantar pressure on the diabetic foot during walking. Med Biol Eng Comput 2008;46(4):363–71.
76. Malakoutikhah H, Madenci E, Latt LD. Evaluation of assumptions in foot and ankle biomechanical models. Clin Biomech 2022;100:105807.

Thermal Injuries Occurring to the Foot: A Review

John M. Tarazi, MD[a,b,*], Adam D. Bitterman, DO[a,b]

KEY WORDS

- Thermal injuries • Foot and ankle • Burn injuries • Frostbite

KEY POINTS

- Thermal injuries are one of the most common injuries in both civilian and combat scenarios.
- This present review examines the: 1) epidemiology; 2) etiology; 3) pathophysiology and classification; and 4) treatment of thermal injuries occurring to the foot.
- This is the first review, to our knowledge, to examine management of thermal injuries occurring to the foot.

INTRODUCTION

According to the World Health Organization, approximately 11 million people in 2004 sustained severe burns requiring medical attention.[1] Unfortunately, with an estimated 265,000 deaths each year resulting from flame burns, this number only rises when accounting for other forms of thermal environmental burn injuries. In addition, the Centers for Disease Control and Prevention (CDC) ranks burns and fires as the third leading cause of death in the home.[2] Based on statistics tabulated by the American Burn Association (ABA), the causes of the thermal burn injuries between 2005 and 2014 in order of prevalence are as follows: (1) flame, (2) scald, (3) contact, (4) electrical, and (5) chemical.[3] Considering that more than 500,000 burn injuries occur in the United States annually, a majority of these injuries do not need to be addressed in a hospital setting and can be treated on an outpatient basis.[3–5]

Burn injuries are traumatic and occur when skin cells or deeper tissues are destroyed by heat, cold, electricity, or caustic chemicals.[3] Even though the foot only encompasses a small percentage of the body, thermal heat burns can be catastrophic. The skin, which consists of the epidermis and dermis, is the largest organ in the body. The thickness of these layers of the skin varies from 0.05 mm on the eyelids to more than 5 mm on the soles of the feet. Variety also exists in the time required to heal a thermal skin burn.

[a] Donald and Barbara Zucker, School of Medicine at Hofstra/Northwell, 500 Hofstra boulevard, Hempstead, NY 11549, USA; [b] Department of Orthopaedic Surgery, Northwell Health—Huntington Hospital, 270 Park Avenue, Huntington, NY 11743, USA
* Corresponding author.
E-mail address: jmtarazi@gmail.com

Foot Ankle Clin N Am 28 (2023) 173–185
https://doi.org/10.1016/j.fcl.2022.12.001
1083-7515/23/© 2022 Elsevier Inc. All rights reserved.

Burns involving the face have a higher density of glands and appendages, which heal at a faster rate with minimal scarring compared with the palmar of plantar surfaces.[6] Furthermore, they are classified based on the depth or extent of tissue injury and can be designated into one of four categories of respective burn depth: (1) superficial; (2) superficial partial thickness; (3) deep partial thickness; and (4) full thickness.

The major goals of treatment of foot burns are the prevention of infection, scar contracture, joint stiffness, and a lengthy healing course. For patients being treated with burn injuries in the hospital setting other complications resulting from the burn injury must be addressed and can include hemodynamic stability, fluid resuscitation, nutritional supplementation, and tests for peripheral circulation. Comorbid conditions such as diabetes, cardiovascular disease, and peripheral vascular disease are risk factors that should be evaluated because they may impede wound healing. The present is a review of the: (1) epidemiology; (2) etiology; (3) pathophysiology and classification; and (4) treatment of thermal injuries occurring to the foot.

EPIDEMIOLOGY

The shear frequency of burn injuries guarantees that every health care professional will treat a burn patient over the course of their career. In 2000, the cost for burn injuries affecting children in the United States surpassed $211 million.[1] Causes of burns vary and include residential fires, automobile accidents, forest fires, chemical burns, abuse, and work related.[7] Gender differences have been reported in evaluating individuals affected by thermal burn injuries. According to the ABA from 2005 to 2014, considering the total number of patients admitted to burn centers, 68% were male, whereas 32% were females. The number of male patients treated for burns injuries in the emergency department from 1993 and 2004 was 50% greater than female patients (270 per 100,000 and 180 per 100,000, respectively).[3] In 2006, the mortality rates for burn deaths in the United States for males and females under the age of 20 were nearly identical (0.7 vs 0.64 per 100,000). The patients admitted to burn centers also differ based on ethnicity. Caucasians presented most frequently, followed by African Americans, Hispanics and, other populations (59%, 20%, 14%, and 7%, respectively).[2]

Burns affecting less than 20% of the total body surface area (TBSA) in children ages 0 to 15 years of age are the fifth most common cause of nonfatal childhood injuries after intracranial injury, open wounds, poisoning, and forearm fractures.[8,9] The frequency of hospital admissions for children with a burn injury globally occurs at a rate of 8 per 100,000, which suggests that the majority of burns in this age population are probably minor scald or contact burns not requiring hospital admission. In 2008, the US rate for nonfatal burns was 156 per 100,000 in children under the age of 18.[10] Two-thirds of children under two years of age are hospitalized for the treatment of burns less than 10% of their TBSA. The elderly population also has a high susceptibility to incur burn injuries, where sixty percent of the elderly population over the age of 60 are hospitalized for burns greater than 10% of their TBSA. Furthermore, the in-hospital mortality rate in burn centers between 1999 and 2008 was 9% for patients in their seventh decade of life, 16% for the eighth, and 20% for patients over the age of 80.[10]

ETIOLOGY

More than 90% of burns can be attributed to carelessness.[9] Prevention of burns is essential, which is why education is paramount, especially in our high-risk populations. Significant improvements in prevention of burn injuries, medical management, and education have been implemented in recent years. The rates of burn deaths in high-income countries have decreased due to improved treatment and care over the past two decades.[11] However, updated prevention protocols and advancements in treatment have not been fully integrated in low-to-middle-income countries across the world. This has resulted in increased disability and mortality. Globally, the majority of deaths from burn injuries (90%) occur in lower-middle or low-income countries.[1,11] Scalds are considered the number one type of burn injury, resulting in greater than 3500 emergency department visits each year.[11] Development of a thermal burn injury is directly proportional to the contact time of water on the skin and the temperature of the water. Water temperature of 65°C to 70°C takes only one second to burn the skin. Comparatively, water temperature of 45°C takes more than 7.5 h of contact time to burn the skin. The most common foot burn affecting children are due to scalds or hot tap water.[7,12] The majority of burns are unintentional; however, from 1999 to 2008, 2% of all admissions to US burns centers were due to child abuse by burning and less than 1% of admissions were for self-inflicted or attempted suicide.[9]

Burns of the feet are serious issues that not only affect children, but also older populations and those with diabetes. Age-related deterioration in coordination, cognition, balance, and judgment correlates with the higher susceptibly to burn injuries. In addition, the elderly affected by thermal burn injuries are also more likely to succumb to infections and metabolic complications.[13] The average TBSA of elderly patients treated for scald burns is 7%; however, the mortality rate in this age group is 22%.[7,9,11] Burn injuries occurring in individuals with comorbid conditions such as diabetes, neuropathy, peripheral vascular disease, and tobacco history tend to result in prolonged healing times, higher incidence of infection and other complications.[14] With decreased or absent sensory feedback in the lower extremities, a person with peripheral neuropathy may not feel the dangerously hot stimulus, in turn increasing the time the skin is in contact with the surface.[7] Diabetic neuropathy is considered to be a significant risk factor for patients sustaining burns to the feet (68% incidence compared with 17% in the nondiabetic control group) as poor healing capabilities can be culprit to nosocomial infections.[15]

Frostbite affects individuals living at higher altitudes, mountain climbing adventurists, and skiers. The complications of frostbite affect parts of the body exposed the elements such as the face and especially the nose. However, as the extremities are furthest away from body's core temperature, the fingers and toes are more prone to frostbite injury and account for 90% of all frostbite injury.[16] With increased participation in winter sports and the rise of homelessness across the country, the civilian population has seen a rise in the amount of frostbite cases.[17] Other risk factors for developing frostbite injuries include: alcohol consumption; psychiatric illness; smoking; homelessness; atherosclerosis; and previous cold weather injury.[17]

PATHOPHYSIOLOGY AND CLASSIFICATION

Thermal injury can cause coagulative necrosis of the epidermis and underlying tissue. The depth of the injury, however, can depend on three key factors: (1) temperature to which the skin is exposed, (2) the specific heat of the causative agent, and (3) the duration of the exposure.

Since burns can be classified into five casual categories (flame, scald, contact, electrical, and chemical) and depths of injury, it is important to understand the pathophysiological changes that occur before assessing treatment options.

Burns

The skin serves as a barrier in the transfer of energy to deeper tissues, however, once the inciting event is eliminated, the response of local tissues can propagate injury to the deeper layers. The depth of burns can vary by the degree of tissue damage and is classified into degree of injury in the epidermis, dermis, subcutaneous fat, and underlying structures. First-degree burns involve the superficial or epidermal layer of skin, as is mostly seen with sunburns. These types of burns do not blister, however, they are considered to be painful, red, and blanch with pressure. Second-degree or partial-thickness burns include the entire epidermis and part of the dermal layer. They can be partial- or full-thickness in depth. These burns blister within 24 h after injury and are painful, red, weeping, and blanch with pressure. Overlap exists when characterizing a second-degree burn. The presentation of a superficial, partial-thickness burn closely resembles first-degree burns, whereas deep, partial-thickness burns more closely resemble full-thickness or third-degree burns. Third-degree or full-thickness burns extend through all layers of the dermis. Subcutaneous tissue can potentially be damaged in these injuries as well. Third-degree burns are typically anesthetic or hypoesthetic because of the destruction of the pain receptor nerve endings. The appearance of third-degree burns can be described as waxy white, leathery gray, or charred black skin known as an eschar. No blisters or blanching with pressure occur with third-degree burns. The deepest burn injury is known as a fourth-degree burn. These burns envelop the deep fascia, muscle, tendons, and potentially bone and are considered life threatening.[5,7]

After evaluation of the burn depth, the next step is to determine the percentage of TBSA burned. When assessing the burn area, it is important to include erythema in the calculation. The Wallace rule of nines divides the body is percentages divisible by nine. For example, the head including the face is 9%, each arm is 9%, the anterior and posterior trunks are each 9%, each leg is 18%, the perineum is 1%, each hand is 1%, and each foot is 1%. Although this classification is commonly used in adults, it is not accurate in the evaluation of burns in children because of the typical disproportionally large head compared with the body. The Lund and Browder chart is a more accurate method for calculating the TBSA affected by a burn injury. One of the beneficial aspects of the Lund and Browder chart is that the surface area fluctuates depending on the patient's age. However, the foot surface area does not change and remains at a constant 3.5% from birth to late adulthood. When determining the percentage of burn area affected, this classification accounts for variation in body shape and age, therefore, it can be used in children.[7,18]

Burns to the foot are considered major burns. Mechanism of injury is essential when evaluating foot burns because it provides insight into the depth of the injury. When a burn patient presents to the emergency department after a trauma, the more life-threatening injury must take precedence. When dealing with a significant traumatic injury, an unintentional delay in care for burn injuries to the foot may result. This negatively affects prognosis of the foot burn because the progression of a burn can potentially increase in depth for up to 72 h after initial burn injury. Once all life-threatening injuries and complications are addressed, attention is then directed to evaluation of the foot burn. Initial evaluation is paramount for the prognosis of foot burns. To initiate appropriate treatment, the clinician must assess the extent of tissue damage to differentiate a superficial burn from partial- and full-thickness burn.[7]

Frostbite

The pathophysiology of frostbite injuries can be broken down into three phases. Phase one includes cooling and freezing. The body initially responds to cold exposure through arterial vasoconstriction and is then followed by Hunting's response that is the body's response to the cooling or freezing skin tissue by alternating cycles of vasoconstriction and vasodilation every 10 minutes. This process attempts to prevent a severe drop in core temperature. As cooling continues, the cold-induced vasodilation (CIVD) response fails and finally pain sensation is lost between 7°C and 9°C. With further cold exposure, extracellular crystals develop resulting in sludging, stasis, and intracellular dehydration. When intracellular ice crystals form and expand, they have the potential of causing mechanical destruction of cell membranes. Phase two of frostbite is rewarming. During this phase, extracellular and intracellular crystals melt and intracellular swelling occurs. Edema and blisters form due to the increased permeability and extravasation of fluid from endothelial cells within capillaries. Phase three of frostbite is progressive tissue injury, where inflammation, vascular stasis, and thromboses lead to ischemia and progressive tissue damage.

The classification system for frostbite injury is divided into four degrees with a progressive depth of injury. Clinically, first-degree frostbite injury includes the formation of a numb central white plaque with surrounding erythema. Second-degree frostbite is characterized by blister formation surrounded by erythema and edema. The blisters are filled with clear or milky fluid in the first 24 h. Third-degree frostbite injury is defined by hemorrhagic blisters which result in black eschars after 2 weeks. The fourth-degree of frostbite includes complete necrosis of skin tissue. An updated classification system divides frostbite into two categories; superficial frostbite and deep frostbite. Superficial frostbite includes first- and second-degree frostbite while deep frostbite includes third- and fourth-degree levels.

TREATMENT
Burns

Treatment of foot burns is determined by the size or percentage of TBSA as well as the depth of the burn. Even though a majority of isolated foot burns can be treated on an outpatient basis, hospital management is beneficial because of early debridement, a clean environment for dressing changes, daily assessment of wound depth, and access to a multispecialty team of health care professionals.[7] Physical therapy is essential in the management of foot burns to initiate early stretching and range of motion exercises.[5,19] Failure to address a thermal injury to the foot with appropriate first-line treatment can lead to serious morbidity. If uncertain as to the treatment protocol for a foot burn, many clinicians err on the side of caution and typically refer the patient to a burn center or hospital for further evaluation and management. This increased attention to patient care is especially beneficial in infants encountering scald injuries. Owing to the infant's much thinner plantar skin compared with that of an adult, they are more susceptible to full-thickness type injuries. For adults succumbing to scald injuries however, admission to a burn center is typically not required since the injury is relatively superficial in nature[7,12]

The initial treatment protocol for foot burns consists of immediate cooling the skin, followed by cleaning and removing debris through debridement. Burn wounds on the foot are treated with sterile, room-temperature or cool water around 12°C for preliminary pain relief. The skin should be cooled for no longer than five minutes to avoid maceration. Alternatively, sterile saline or cool water-soaked gauze around 12°C can be applied to the burn wound for up to 30 minutes until debridement and the eventual dressings are applied.[20,21] After cooling the skin, the foot burn should be cleaned using soap and tap water. This process can be extremely painful for the patient and it is recommended that a local or regional anesthetic block is instituted before cleansing the wound. During the hospital course, it is recommended to manage pain of superficial burns with nonsteroidal anti-inflammatories (NSAIDs) and opioids. Deeper foot burns involving the epidermis can initially be managed with intravenous medications such as morphine with a pain management physician closely involved with care. Elevation of the lower extremity and foot above the level of the heart can also help to reduce pain, inflammation, and edema.[21–23] Antiseptic disinfectants such as Hibiclens (chlorhexidine gluconate solution) and Betadine (povidone-iodine solution) should be avoided in foot burn wounds since they can potentially inhibit the healing process.[5,19,24] Before application of the wound dressing, all necrotic, sloughed, and devitalized tissue should be debrided. Mechanical debridement is performed using brushing, scraping, and/or curetting.[21] Burn blisters that are ruptured should be debrided and cleansed before adding a dressing. However, controversy exists regarding treatment of intact, clean burn blisters and unfortunately no standard treatment protocol exists. Some clinicians argue that leaving the roof of a blister intact acts a skin barrier against infection, whereas others claim an increased risk of infection exists if the blister is not debrided due to the increased number of vasoconstrictive and inflammatory mediators. Leaving a blister intact has the potential of impeding accurate diagnosis of burn depth.[7,25] Aspiration of an intact blister should not be performed with a needle because of the increased risk of infection.[26] If purulent or discolored fluid exists within the blister, many clinicians recommend de-roofing the blister, especially if it overlies extensor and flexor surfaces such as joints, which can hinder range of motion.[25–27] Treatment and healing times vary for each degree of foot burn injuries. First-degree burns are the typically self-limiting as they are usually able to heal with minimal to no medical intervention. Moisturizing lotions, emollients, and basic burn dressings such as antimicrobial ointments and nonadherent gauze can be used along with supportive are. The healing time for a first-degree burn is about 3 to 7 days in duration. The treatment options for second-degree burns differ based on the extent of burn depth. The superficial, partial-thickness foot burns are treated similarly to first-degree burns and include: supportive care, observation, and daily dressing changes consisting of antimicrobial agents such as bacitracin or silver sulfadiazine with nonadherent gauze including Adaptic (non-adhering silicone; 3M, Minnesota, USA) or xeroform (3% bismuth tribromophenate) dressing. Silver sulfadiazine (SSD) is the most commonly used topical antimicrobial in burn wounds due to its effectiveness in preventing infection, however, it does have some drawbacks. Silver sulfadiazine can only be used as a superficial antimicrobial agent since it is unable to penetrate deep into a burn wound or scar. One side effect of SSD is cytotoxicity to epithelial cells, which results in inhibiting wound healing. Therefore, SSD should be stopped immediately upon visualization of healthy epithelial budding.[5,7] Women who are pregnant or breastfeeding and infants under two months of age should not be treated with SSD because of the risk of neural damage from sulfonamide kernicterus.[28] Another frequently used antimicrobial agent in burn wounds is mafenide acetate. Advantages of mafenide acetate are that it can penetrate deep into burn eschars and prevent bacterial colonization of the wound, therefore controlling commonly seen infections with burns such as *Pseudomonas aeruginosa*. Some disadvantages of mafenide acetate include the potential pain caused to the patient during application to superficial, partial-thickness burns and a link between this product and metabolic acidosis.[7] Honey-based wound care products are also effective in healing superficial, partial-thickness burn wounds. Furthermore, Boekema and colleagues[29] and Jull and colleagues[30] showed that honey-based dressings are able to heal partial-thickness burns quicker than conventional dressings such as polyurethane film, paraffin gauze, and soframycin-impregnated gauze. Wet, weeping second-degree burn wounds require drying agents. DuoDERM (ConvaTec, Deeside, UK) is a hydrocolloid dressing, composed of gelatin and polymers, which not only provides adequate coverage over the wound, but also forms a gel when activated by wound exudate.[31] Dressings containing silver are also beneficial in addressing burn wound exudate. As mentioned earlier, silver has excellent broad-spectrum antimicrobial coverage. Common examples include Acquacel (ConvaTec, Deeside, UK) and Acticoat (Smith & Nephew, London, UK) dressings that are comprised of nanocrystalline silver. These silver dressings allow the continuous release of silver into the burn wound, preventing biofilms and bacterial growth. Furthermore, the dressings are able to remain on the patient's wound for 5 to 7 days in duration.[7,32] The body's natural healing process sends keratinocytes found within sweat glands and hair follicles that aid the regeneration process in burn wounds.[5,33]

More extensive treatment must be implemented when dealing with deep, partial-thickness burns and third-degree or full-thickness burns. The burn eschar must first be excised with sharp debridement, through cutting or curettage, followed by coverage of the wound. Burn eschars can be excised to the layer of the deep fascia, known as an escharotomy, or shaved superficially with a tangential excision. In some circumstances, a fasciotomy may need to be performed with burn injuries. This a limb salvage type of procedure performed in the emergency setting to treat acute compartment syndrome. A fasciotomy is used to incise the fascia, in turn, relieving pressures within one of the compartments of the leg or foot. There are a variety of surgical treatment options that can be used in the treatment of full-thickness burn wounds. Primary goals of care include immediate wound coverage, increasing the rate of wound healing, reducing the inflammatory response, and reducing scarring. Wound coverage can be achieved through skin grafts and skin substitutes. The most common plastic surgery technique for wound coverage is using a skin graft, which can include the use of an autograft, allograft, or xenograft. These options have proven to be successful in management of a deep full-thickness burn wounds. Skin grafts, which can be split- or full-thickness, are able to revascularize burn wounds by promoting angiogenesis through the process of capillary ingrowth in the wound bed. To minimize infection and blood loss, timing is also essential as the decision to graft a burn wound should be performed within 5 days of injury. Harvesting a skin graft from the patient's donor site for a split- or full-thickness autograft is performed with a dermatome and is best obtained from uninjured skin. The skin graft is then typically meshed to increase graft take and prevent hematoma and infection.

Two main categories exist when defining skin substitutes: single-layer and composite skin substitutes.[34] Single-layer skin substitutes are dermal substitutes that can be applied to deep, full-thickness wound deficits before application of a skin graft. They include, but are not limited to, human dermal matrix and bovine collagen sheet. These dermal skin substitutes facilitate wound epithelialization and assist with increasing granulation tissue. Composite skin substitutes consist of bioengineered synthetic skin substitutes. Bioengineered synthetic skin substitutes allow for ingrowth of blood vessels, fibroblasts, and wound coverage by epithelial cells, however, growth factors and matrix components can be synthetically added to the skin substitutes to enhance the effectiveness of these products.[7,34–38]

Deeper burn wounds increase the likelihood of exposing tendons in the foot. Unfortunately, these patients require more extensive surgical intervention including a local or free flap. These types of procedures on the foot are considered more compromising compared with other parts of the body Reconstruction of the foot can be achieved through a number of different local musculofascial flaps. Dorsalis pedis artery fascio-cutaneous flaps are used for ankle coverage. A reversed dorsalis pedis artery flap can be used for coverage over the distal foot and great toe. The distal foot, web spaces, and toes can also be resurfaced using the first dorsal metatarsal artery flap. The extensor digitorum brevis flap is supplied from the lateral tarsal artery and provides coverage for burn wounds involving the toes to the distal tibia. Plantar skin flaps are constructed to transfer healthy skin from the non-weight-bearing aspect of the foot to the plantar weight-bearing aspect of the sole of the foot. The medial plantar flap from the medial plantar artery is composed of glabrous skin and has the ability of rotating to cover heel defects up to 7 cm in diameter. A various number of other local flaps exist derived from the abductor hallucis, abductor digiti minimi, and flexor digitorum brevis muscles. Preoperative evaluation is crucial when considering a flap surgical procedure. This can be achieved through noninvasive vascular testing to assess for patency and healing potential. Patency of the anterior tibial and dorsalis pedis arteries is required for proximally based flaps whereas distally based flaps require patency of the posterior tibial artery and plantar vessels.

When considering performing split-thickness skin grafts or free flaps, the benefits of early excision with grafting result in faster healing times among burn patients. Even if debridement or excision is not performed, foot burns can still take 3 to 6 weeks for the eschar to separate from the healthy skin underneath and another 2 to 3 weeks for skin graft incorporation and final wound healing. It is never recommended to delay treatment when dealing with foot burns. Early excision and skin grafting decreases stress, hypermetabolism, bacterial load, necrotic, and nonviable burn tissue, which can prevent against a potential source of sepsis.

Staphylococcus aureus has been found to be the most common organism found in the wound after a burn injury, followed by streptococci.[39] To reduce the incidence of infection, prophylactic broad-spectrum antibiotics are recommended for most foot burn injuries treated either in the hospital or outpatient setting[7,12,40,41]

The soft tissues and skin of plantar surface of the foot contain shock absorption properties, allowing cushioning and protection to the underlying musculature and bony surfaces.

When the plantar surface of the foot is burned, this anatomy can be extremely difficult to recreate. After a plantar foot burn injury, the bottom of the foot will no longer be as robust or resilient against the constant repetitive loading forces and microtrauma that is faced on a daily basis. Comparisons of split- or full-thickness skin grafts and flaps with respect to the weight-bearing surface have shown no difference among these treatment modalities.[7] After skin graft or flap procedures, patients tend to avoid weight-bearing resurfaced areas of the plantar foot. Ultimately, abnormal gait patterns develop among these patients, including shorter ground contact time and decreased load on the affected foot during the stance phase of gait. Patient education and postoperative management are essential after skin graft and flap procedures. Custom orthotics and custom orthopedic shoes should be implemented to maintain long-term success with the reconstructed skin surface. Skin grafts and free flaps are great options to cover affected foot burn surface, but chronic recurrent ulceration is a serious problem affecting patients. Recurrent ulceration on the plantar foot must be addressed in a timely manner to avoid further long-term complications.[7] The foot and ankle surgeon must not only be capable of dealing with chronic nonhealing recurrent ulcerations, but also cognizant of potential malignant changes occurring in long-standing ulcerations.[40] Marjolin's ulcer is a chronic ulcerations that can undergo malignant transitions into squamous cell carcinoma.[42] Therefore, it is important to have burn scars routinely evaluated and chronic recurrent ulcerations treated immediately.[7,21,43]

Other problems associated with foot burns are hypertrophic scars and contracture of the toes or ankle.[44] During the healing process, the body increases production of vascular ingrowth, fibroblasts, collagen, edema, and interstitial deposition within the burn wound. This results in environment conducive to the formation of hypertrophic scarring and skin contracture. One important factor contributing to hypertrophic scarring is time. When the epithelialization process for burn wound healing takes longer than 2 weeks to heal, one-third of the newly healed skin becomes hypertrophic. Scars will develop after 3 weeks of epithelialization in 78% of the burn sites. Toe burn scar contractures result in significant difficulties with performing activities of daily living, as well as functional limitations, and inability to wear standard shoe gear. Difficulty ambulating and joint pain increases with more severe toe contractures, which results in further subsequent trauma and injury. Scarring leading to toe contractures is more prevalent among growing children.[45] As children develop, the scar contracture remains stagnant, whereas the soft tissues surrounding the scar continue to grow resulting in further contracture of the scar. If not appropriately treated, permanent functional and skeletal deformities may develop. Skin contractures are especially evident with burn injuries to the dorsum of the foot which cause hyperextension of the toes and metatarsophalangeal joint subluxation. The skin on the dorsum of the foot is extremely thin which may result in the possible exposure of tendons with foot burns as well. When performing an escharotomy in these patients, it is vital for the surgeon to be conscientious and meticulous when performing the debridement to preserve the paratenon around each exposed tendon.[46] This careful dissection technique will favor the addition of a split-thickness skin graft and will hopefully prevent toe contractures. Prevention of toe contractures after foot burns involve splinting the toes while educating the patient on proper shoe gear to maintain the toes in an anatomically rectus position. If conservative management and prevention of toe contractures fails, surgical treatment must be rendered. Surgical options for toe contractures first involve release of scar bands. Local tissue rearrangement is performed using the Z-plasty technique when scars cross-relaxed skin tension lines or create syndactyly in the web space between toes. When tendons are under significant tension, tenotomies, tendon lengthening, and capsulotomies are performed to address contracted extensor tendons located on the dorsum of the foot. Mallet or hammer toe deformities may be treated with an arthrodesis or arthroplasty procedure. Pin fixation can hold the rearranged bony structures in correct anatomical alignment for about 4 weeks in duration before removal. Postoperative care is critical to prevent toe contracture recurrence. Moisturizing lotions and creams are applied to scars along with compression garments to prevent hypertrophic scarring. Immobilization during the immediate postoperative healing course is proceeded by progressive physical therapy that improves functional mobility and toe position.[7,47–50]

Frostbite

Treatment of frostbite is constantly undergoing new protocols. However, treatment of immediate acute frostbite injury has remained unchanged. Traditional first-line treatment involves removing the individual from the cold thermal environment, which is a priority. Once the cold insult has been removed, assessing for hypothermia is crucial and requires immediate attention. Immediately after providing intravenous fluids and monitoring vitals, rapid rewarming of tissues of the affected body part includes using water temperatures at 40°C to 42°C. When making the determination if a toe or limb is salvageable from gangrene due to tissue necrosis, the clinician must wait for demarcation over the next several months before considering amputation. Many adjunctive therapies have developed over the years to combat frostbite injuries of the feet. These treatment modalities include low-molecular-weight dextran, anticoagulants such as heparin, vasodilators such as reserpine, thrombolytic agents such as tPA, antibiotics, ibuprofen to inhibit harmful prostaglandins, tetanus prophylaxis, and hyperbaric oxygen therapy.[16,51–53] Although more studies are needed to further support advancements in this topic, these aforementioned treatments have garnered much support by various foot and ankle and emergency specialists.

SUMMARY

Thermal injuries are a major cause of worldwide morbidity and mortality with lifelong and debilitating injuries that can have serious psychological and economic implications. In this review, the authors examine the (1) epidemiology, (2) etiology, (3) pathophysiology and classification, and (4) treatment of thermal injuries occurring to the foot. Owing to the paucity of recent literature, future studies should involve more prospective and retrospective studies assessing each of the treatment modalities for all types of thermal injuries. This article should serve as a guide for orthopedic surgeons and emergency physicians when addressing patients presenting with thermal injuries to the foot and ankle.

CLINICS CARE POINTS

- Based on statistics tabulated by the American Burn Association (ABA), the causes of the thermal burn injuries between 2005-2014 in order of prevalence are: 1) flame; 2) scald; 3) contact; 4) electrical; and 5) chemical.

- Considering that more than 500,000 burn injuries occur in the United States annually, a majority of these injuries do not need to be addressed in a hospital setting and can be treated on an outpatient basis.

- Burns are classified based on the depth or extent of tissue injury and can be designated into one of four categories of respective burn depth: 1) superficial; 2) superficial partial thickness; 3) deep partial thickness; and 4) full thickness.

- Even though many isolated foot burns can be treated on an outpatient basis, hospital management is beneficial because of early debridement, a clean environment for dressing changes, daily assessment of wound depth, and access to a multispecialty team of health care professionals.

- Physical therapy is essential in the management of foot burns in order to initiate early stretching and range of motion exercises. Failure to address a thermal injury to the foot with appropriate first line treatment can lead to serious morbidity.

- The initial treatment protocol for foot burns consists of immediate cooling the skin, followed by cleaning and removing debris through debridement. Deeper foot burns can initially be managed with intravenous medications such as morphine with a pain management physician closely involved with care.

- Treatment for frostbite is constantly undergoing new protocols, however, treatment for immediate acute frostbite injury has remained unchanged. Traditional first line treatmentinvolves removing the individual from the cold thermal environment, which is a priority. Immediately after providing intravenous fluids and monitoring vitals, rapid rewarming of tissues of the affected body part includes using water temperatures at 40-42°C. Adjunctive therapies have included low-molecular weight dextran, anticoagulants such as heparin, vasodilators such as reserpine, thrombolytic agents such as tPA, antibiotics, ibuprofen to inhibit harmful prostaglandins, tetanus prophylaxis, and hyperbaric oxygen therapy.

REFERENCES

1. World Health Organization n.d, Available at: https://www.who.int. Accessed December 1, 2021.

2. American Burn Association–Fact Sheet n.d, Available at: https://ameriburn.org/who-we-are/media/burn-incidence-fact-sheet/. Accessed December 1, 2021.

3. American Burn Association n.d, Available at: https://ameriburn.org. Accessed December 1, 2021.

4. Warner PM, Coffee TL, Yowler CJ. Outpatient burn management. Surg Clin North Am 2014. https://doi.org/10.1016/j.suc.2014.05.009.

5. Mertens DM, Jenkins ME, Warden GD. Outpatient burn management. Nurs Clin North Am 1997.

6. American Society of Plastic Surgeons n.d. Available at: https://www.plasticsurgery.org.

7. Shah BR. Burns of the feet. Clin Podiatr Med Surg 2002;19(1):109–23.

8. Centers for Disease Control and Prevention n.d, Available at: https://www.cdc.gov/safechild/images/cdc-childhoodinjury.pdf. Accessed December 1, 2021.

9. Peck MD. Epidemiology of burns throughout the world. Part I: distribution and risk factors. Burns 2011. https://doi.org/10.1016/j.burns.2011.06.005.

10. Jeschke MG, Kamolz LP, Sjöberg F, et al. Handbook of burns: acute burn care 2012;1. https://doi.org/10.1007/978-3-7091-0348-7.

11. Runyan CW, Johnson RM, Yang J, et al. Risk and protective factors for fires, burns, and carbon monoxide poisoning in U.S. households. Am J Prev Med 2005. https://doi.org/10.1016/j.amepre.2004.09.014.

12. Hemington-Gorse S, Pellard S, Wilson-Jones N, et al. Foot burns: Epidemiology and management. Burns 2007. https://doi.org/10.1016/j.burns.2006.11.014.

13. Mabrouk A, Maher A, Nasser S. An epidemiologic study of elderly burn patients in Ain Shams University Burn Unit, Cairo, Egypt. Burns 2003. https://doi.org/10.1016/S0305-4179(03)00071-8.

14. Geerlings SE, Hoepelman AIM. Immune dysfunction in patients with diabetes mellitus (DM). FEMS Immunol Med Microbiol 1999. https://doi.org/10.1016/S0928-8244(99)00142-X.

15. Memmel H, Kowal-Vern A, Latenser BA. Infections in diabetic burn patients. Diabetes Care 2004. https://doi.org/10.2337/diacare.27.1.229.

16. Handford C, Buxton P, Russell K, et al. Frostbite: a practical approach to hospital management. Extrem Physiol Med 2014. https://doi.org/10.1186/2046-7648-3-7.

17. Basit H., Wallen T.J. and Dudley C., Frostbite. [Updated 2021 Nov 5]. In: StatPearls [Internet]. Treasure Island (FL): StatPearls Publishing, 2022. Available at: https://www.ncbi.nlm.nih.gov/books/NBK536914/n.d. Accessed December 1, 2021.

18. Hettiaratchy S, Papini R. Initial management of a major burn: II—assessment and resuscitation. BMJ 2004. https://doi.org/10.1136/bmj.329.7457.101.

19. Baxter CR. Management of burn wounds. Dermatol Clin 1993. https://doi.org/10.1016/s0733-8635(18)30223-7.

20. Pushkar NS, Sandorminsky BP. Cold treatment of burns. Burns 1982. https://doi.org/10.1016/0305-4179(82)90056-0.

21. Hartford CE. Care of outpatient burns. Fourth Ed. Total Burn Care; 2012. https://doi.org/10.1016/B978-1-4377-2786-9.00006-0.

22. Summer GJ, Puntillo KA, Miaskowski C, et al. Burn injury pain: the continuing challenge. J Pain 2007. https://doi.org/10.1016/j.jpain.2007.02.426.

23. Ulmer JF. Burn pain management: a guideline-based approach. J Burn Care Rehabil 1988;19(2):151–9.

24. Greenhalgh DG. The healing of burn wounds. Dermatol Nurs 1996. https://doi.org/10.1016/s0094-1298(20)30546-0.

25. Sargent RL. Management of blisters in the partial-thickness burn: an integrative research review. J Burn Care Res 2006. https://doi.org/10.1097/01.bcr. 0000191961.95907.b1.

26. Waitzman AA, Neligan PC. How to manage burns in primary care. Can Fam Physician 1993.

27. Rockwell WB, Ehrlich HP. Should burn blister fluid be evacuated? J Burn Care Rehabil 1990. https://doi.org/10.1097/00004630-199001000-00020.

28. Peate WF. Outpatient management of burns. Am Fam Physician 1992;45: 1321–30.

29. Boekema BKHL, Pool L, Ulrich MMW. The effect of a honey based gel and silver sulphadiazine on bacterial infections of in vitro burn wounds. Burns 2013. https://doi.org/10.1016/j.burns.2012.09.008.

30. Jull AB, Cullum N, Dumville JC, et al. Honey as a topical treatment for wounds. Cochrane Database Syst Rev 2015. https://doi.org/10.1002/14651858. CD005083.pub4.

31. Wyatt D, Mc Gowan DN, Najarian MP. Comparison of a hydrocolloid dressing and silver sulfadiazine cream in the outpatient management of second-degree burns. J Trauma - Inj Infect Crit Care 1990. https://doi.org/10.1097/00005373-199007000-00016.

32. Dunn K, Edwards-Jones V. The role of ActicoatTM with nanocrystalline silver in the management of burns. Burns 2004. https://doi.org/10.1016/S0305-4179(04) 90000-9.

33. Papini R. ABC of burns: management of burn injuries of various depths. Br Med J 2004. https://doi.org/10.1136/bmj.329.7458.158.

34. Halim AS, Khoo TL, Shah SJ. Biologic and synthetic skin substitutes: an overview. Indian J Plast Surg 2010. https://doi.org/10.4103/0970-0358.70712.

35. Alharbi Z, Piatkowski A, Dembinski R, et al. Treatment of burns in the first 24 hours: simple and practical guide by answering 10 questions in a step-by-step form. World J Emerg Surg 2012. https://doi.org/10.1186/1749-7922-7-13.

36. Frink M, Hildebrand F, Krettek C, et al. Compartment syndrome of the lower leg and foot. Clin Orthop Relat Res 2010. https://doi.org/10.1007/s11999-009-0891-x.

37. Ferreira MC, Paggiaro AO, Isaac C, et al. Skin substitutes: current concepts and a new classification system Substitutos cutâneos: conceitos atuais e proposta de classificação. Rev Bras Cir Plast 2011;26(4):696–702.

38. Capla JM, Ceradini DJ, Tepper OM, et al. Skin graft vascularization involves precisely regulated regression and replacement of endothelial cells through both angiogenesis and vasculogenesis. Plast Reconstr Surg 2006. https://doi.org/10. 1097/01.prs.0000201459.91559.7f.

39. Norbury W, Herndon DN, Tanksley J, et al. Infection in burns. Surg Infect (Larchmt) 2016. https://doi.org/10.1089/sur.2013.134.

40. Gore D, Desai M, Herndon DN, et al. Comparison of complications during rehabilitation between conservative and early surgical management in thermal burns involving the feet of children and adolescents. J Burn Care Rehabil 1988. https://doi.org/10.1097/00004630-198801000-00024.

41. Trent JT, Kirsner RS. Wounds and malignancy. Adv Skin Wound Care 2003. https://doi.org/10.1097/00129334-200301000-00014.

42. Copcu E, Aktas A, Şişman N, et al. Thirty-one cases of Marjolin's ulcer. Clin Exp Dermatol 2003. https://doi.org/10.1046/j.1365-2230.2003.01210.x.

43. Sabin SR, Goldstein G, Rosenthal HG, et al. Aggressive squamotous cell carcinoma originating as a marjolin's ulcer. Dermatol Surg 2004. https://doi.org/10.1111/j.1524-4725.2004.30072.x.

44. Ong SL, Bajuri MY, Abdul Suki MH, et al. Hypertrophic scar with contracture over the fourth toe secondary to snake bite wound: to salvage or amputate? Cureus 2020. https://doi.org/10.7759/cureus.9451.

45. Alison WF, Moore MI, Reilly DA, et al. Reconstruction of foot burn contractures in children. J Burn Care Rehabil 1993. https://doi.org/10.1097/00004630-199301000-00009.

46. Zhang L., Labib A. and Hughes P.G., Escharotomy. [Updated 2021 Oct 27]. In: StatPearls [Internet]. Treasure Island (FL): StatPearls Publishing, 2022. Available at: https://www.ncbi.nlm.nih.gov/books/NBK482120/n.d. Accessed December 1, 2021.

47. Helm PA. Burn rehabilitation: Dimensions of the problem. Clin Plast Surg 1992. https://doi.org/10.1016/s0094-1298(20)30942-1.

48. Kucan JO, Bash D. Reconstruction of the burned foot. Clin Plast Surg 1992.

49. Deitch EA, Wheelahan TM, Rose MP, et al. Hypertrophic burn scars: Analysis of variables. J Trauma - Inj Infect Crit Care 1983. https://doi.org/10.1097/00005373-198310000-00009.

50. Chang JB, Kung TA, Levi B, et al. Surgical management of burn flexion and extension contractures of the toes. J Burn Care Res 2014. https://doi.org/10.1097/BCR.0b013e3182a368fc.

51. Bruen KJ, Ballard JR, Morris SE, et al. Reduction of the incidence of amputation in frostbite injury with thrombolytic therapy. Arch Surg 2007. https://doi.org/10.1001/archsurg.142.6.546.

52. Jones LM, Coffey RA, Natwa MP, et al. The use of intravenous tPA for the treatment of severe frostbite. Burns 2017. https://doi.org/10.1016/j.burns.2017.01.013.

53. Kemper TCPM, De Jong VM, Anema HA, et al. Frostbite of both first digits of the foot treated with delayed hyperbaric oxygen: a case report and review of literature. Undersea Hyperb Med 2014;41(1):65–70.

Moving?

Make sure your subscription moves with you!

To notify us of your new address, find your **Clinics Account Number** (located on your mailing label above your name), and contact customer service at:

Email: journalscustomerservice-usa@elsevier.com

800-654-2452 (subscribers in the U.S. & Canada)
314-447-8871 (subscribers outside of the U.S. & Canada)

Fax number: 314-447-8029

Elsevier Health Sciences Division
Subscription Customer Service
3251 Riverport Lane
Maryland Heights, MO 63043

*To ensure uninterrupted delivery of your subscription, please notify us at least 4 weeks in advance of move.

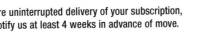

Printed and bound by CPI Group (UK) Ltd, Croydon, CR0 4YY

08/05/2025

01864715-0005